An Executive Guide to Case Management Strategies

Marjorie A. Satinsky, M.A., M.B.A., F.A.C.H.E.

AHA books are published by American Hospital Publishing, Inc., an American Hospital Association company

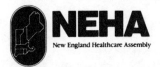

New England Healthcare Assembly

The views expressed in this publication are strictly those of the author and do not necessarily represent official positions of the American Hospital Association or the New England Healthcare Assembly.

Library of Congress Cataloging-in-Publication Data

Satinsky, Marjorie, A.
   An executive guide to case management strategies / Marjorie A. Satinsky.
   Satinsky.
      p.   cm.
   Includes bibliographical references and index.
   ISBN 1-55648-128-4
   1. Hospitals—Case management services. 2. Managed care plans (Medical care). 3. Hospitals—United States—Case management services—Case studies. I. Title.
   [DNLM: 1. Managed Care Programs—organization & administration—United States. W 275 AA1 S2e 1995]
   RA975.5.C36S28   1995
   362.1—dc20
   DNLM/DLC
   for Library of Congress   94-37461
                                                   CIP

Catalog no. 027102

©1995 by American Hospital Publishing, Inc.,
an American Hospital Association company

Printed in the USA

Text set in Goudy
2.5M—2/95—0390
2M—4/96—0438

Linda Conheady, Acquisitions/Development Editor
Anne Hermann, Production Editor
Peggy DuMais, Production Coordinator
Cheryl Kusek, Cover Designer
Marcia Bottoms, Books Division Assistant Director
Brian Schenk, Books Division Director

Contents

List of Figures

About the Author

Marjorie A. Satinsky, M.A., M.B.A., F.A.C.H.E., is director, managed care contracting and operations, Duke Health Network, Duke University Medical Center, Durham, North Carolina. She was formerly in charge of managed care strategy and operations at The Malden Hospital, Malden, Massachusetts, and has assisted other hospitals and physicians with managed care projects. She is a frequent lecturer on managed care at the national, state, and local levels. Ms. Satinsky is a graduate of the Wharton School at the University of Pennsylvania, Philadelphia, and of Brown University, Providence, Rhode Island.

Preface

Changes in the financing and delivery of health care are occurring faster than those of us in the field ever imagined possible. We have known for many years that we needed to confront the issues of access to care, cost, quality, employer-based insurance, and rationing of resources. The 1993 Clinton health care reform proposal challenged all of us, regardless of where we live, to look quickly and carefully for solutions to these difficult problems.

Given the heterogeneity that characterizes the United States, state and local variation in response to major health care issues comes as no surprise. Many regions already have moved, or soon will move, toward an integrated financing and delivery system model, where physicians, facilities, and payers become partners in a single system. For geographic and economic reasons, however, all communities will not experience integration.

Where they do occur, the processes of integration and consolidation will evolve over time. During the transition, it is important that practitioners not lose sight of our ultimate purpose—to take care of patients. We do not have to wait for complete integration to manage patient care in new ways. We can begin to replace what we do now with a more comprehensive case management approach to managing the clinical and financial aspects of care.

Historically, the term *case management* has had many meanings and applications. Commonly used terms like *nursing case management* and *home care case management* emphasize the care giver or the location of care, rather than the mobilization of resources around the patient. Despite this ambiguity of definition, there have been numerous success stories. Case management programs have reduced length of stay, improved treatment and outcomes, and facilitated appropriate resource utilization. Even so, very few programs have realized their full potential—to assist providers and the integrated financing and delivery systems of which they may be a part so as to manage health maintenance and treatment for a defined population.

This book is directed toward two groups of people: those who will establish case management programs and those who will perform the tasks. It is also a resource for those who work in settings where case management already exists.

The impetus for the book was both professional and personal. To strengthen its readiness for managed care, The Malden Hospital (Malden, Massachusetts) developed and implemented case management in the fall of 1992. Within 18 months, the new program had made a measurable impact on patient care, costs, and physician and patient satisfaction. Physicians in the facility's independent practice organization (IPA) enhanced the program by adding an essential medical component. Case management became an organizational approach, not a departmental focus, and the problem-solving orientation of the case managers began to influence many aspects of the delivery system. The research done for this book assisted The Malden Hospital to accelerate the development of the case management approach.

Two personal experiences convinced me of the importance of extending case management beyond the walls of hospitals and other health care institutions. My uncle, a New York resident, was diagnosed with cancer and traveled to Massachusetts for treatment. Access to high-quality clinical care was not the issue. The challenge was the coordination of the medical, financial, and psychosocial aspects of his illness. My own back surgery and determination to return to personally acceptable activities of daily living and athletic enjoyment made me acutely aware of the frustrating lack of coordination between health education, inpatient and outpatient care, and rehabilitation.

For professional and personal reasons, this book came to be. I hope it provides guidance to health care professionals who have the vision to make changes and the courage to apply creative solutions to long-standing problems.

Acknowledgments

Special thanks go to the following at The Malden Hospital: Stanley J. Krygowski, president; Gerald F. O'Neill, treasurer; Robert G. Rulison, executive vice-president; Evelyn M. Soldano, director of case management; Elizabeth Fitzpayne, librarian; Sandra Hamilton, managed care/Malden IPA office; Lyle G. Bohlman, M.D., IPA president; Richard A. Hochman, M.D., IPA medical director; the board of Malden IPA; and the case management department.

Linda H. Conheady, acquisitions and development editor in the Books Division of American Hospital Publishing, Inc.; Susan B. Keener, Sue Keener Associates; and Liz Kramer, New England Healthcare Assembly provided invaluable substantive and editorial suggestions.

I would also like to thank many other supportive colleagues whose observations, insights, and encouragement made this book a reality: Robert Ellertsen, Newton, Massachusetts; Robert S. Galvin, M.D., manager of health care management and medical services, General Electric Aircraft Engines, Lynn, Massachusetts; Jeanne M. Holland, vice-president, managed care and physician services, Beverly Hospital, Beverly, Massachusetts; Amy S. MacNulty, principal, The Bristol Group, Boston; Frank P. Morse III, M.D., chief of surgery, Salem Hospital, Salem, Massachusetts; Andrew H. Nighswander, Health Care Spectrum, Inc., Marblehead, Massachusetts; Cynthia N. Roache, nursing quality assurance coordinator, Wentworth-Douglass Hospital, Dover, New Hampshire; Buzz Satinsky, Esq., Fox, Rothschild, O'Brien and Frankel, Philadelphia; Marva Serotkin, executive director, Cura Visiting Nurses Association, Plymouth, Massachusetts; Neil S. Shore, M.D., president, medical staff, Salem Hospital; and David Wright, Esq., assistant to the senior vice-president for financial services and legal counsel, Salem Hospital.

Introduction

Health care in the 1990s is radically different from what most of us have known. Many of the long-standing problems (for example, access, cost, coverage, and resource allocation) have been, or will be, addressed at regional, state, and, ultimately, national levels. Those who pay the bills—employers, insurers, and employee health and welfare funds—are pressuring providers to provide quality care at more affordable prices.

As the health care system undergoes dramatic transformation, it is easy to lose perspective and to concentrate on action words like *merger, consolidation, re-engineering*, and *downsizing*. Restructuring health care financing and delivery systems will succeed only if patients benefit. Case management is an approach to the clinical and financial management of care that concentrates on patients.

This book was written for multiple audiences. It is a blueprint for professionals who will conceptualize and establish case management within their organizations. For those who will perform the job of case management on a day-to-day basis, it is a handbook with practical suggestions and justification for a new approach. For those who work in settings where case management already exists, it offers an overall framework and ideas for program enhancement.

The first four chapters deal with the what, why, and how of case management. Chapter 1 provides a working definition of the term and suggests some short-term and long-term goals. It describes the variety of applications of the term *case management* that give rise to confusion about what it is and how it operates. Finally, the chapter enumerates the activities that case managers perform, regardless of setting.

Chapter 2 looks at the current health care environment and explains important concepts such as managed care, community care networks, integrated financing and delivery systems, and transitional strategies. It describes the generic elements of health care reform and current approaches of public and private payers and health plans. The chapter also discusses the increasing pressure for provider accountability and the new role hospitals will play in a changing environment.

Chapter 3 offers suggestions for setting up case management. Specific topics deal with introducing the concept of case management, developing a multidisciplinary program, clarifying the definition of case management, sequencing the steps in setting up a program, ensuring evolutionary program development, planning organizational structure and staffing, applying case management beyond the acute care setting, asking the right questions, measuring the impact of case management, and delineating systems for internal and external communications and marketing.

Chapter 4 covers common obstacles that stand in the way of developing case management and suggests strategies for addressing each problem. Barriers such as turf issues, failure to grasp the subtleties surrounding the changing health care environment, passive response to externally set standards, a focus on tools instead of ultimate goals, ineffective reporting relationships, information inadequacies, leadership and accountability deficiencies, conflicting physician issues, operational policies and procedures that impede case management, looking for the magic solution, and systems-specific problems all are addressed in the chapter.

Chapters 5 through 8 comprise four case study examples of case management programs already under way. Chapter 5 describes a program at The Malden Hospital, a 200-bed community institution whose case management effort began in the inpatient acute setting and rapidly expanded. The example shows that development of case management is a process, not an act, and that a multidisciplinary approach is most effective.

Chapter 6 describes an ambulatory-based program in a systems setting at the Friendly Hills HealthCare Network. The role of the geriatric case manager is described in detail.

Chapter 7 describes an innovative model in place at Carondelet St. Mary's Hospital and Health Center, where nurse case managers provide and coordinate care in an ambulatory setting. The involvement of the case management network in a Medicare risk contract is also described.

Chapter 8 delineates the approach to case management taken by Sharp HealthCare, an integrated financing and delivery system.

Chapter 9 illustrates the way in which a system care management program can evolve from case management initiatives established at one of the system components. Lutheran General provides the backdrop for this discussion.

The book provides four appendixes for additional resources. Appendix A contains a suggested curriculum for case managers that can be used as a model. Appendix B describes 14 program-specific features of organizations that already have developed case management programs. It is a good research source for anyone charged with setting up or refining a case management program. Appendix C offers suggestions for selecting a consultant when undertaking case management design and implementation. Appendix D lists the names of individuals contacted at various organizations who provided information for this book.

Finally, at the back of the book there is an index. It will help the reader search for specific information more expediently.

What Is Case Management?

Given the fast-paced change occurring in the health care environment in terms of financing and delivery, it is possible that new methods of organizing, providing, and paying for care will create confusion among the population expected to benefit from the change. As health care organizations and services are combined and reshaped, and as methods of payment encourage less instead of more use of the health care system, health care professionals have an opportunity to ease the transition by means of applying a case management approach to service delivery.

Chapter 1 provides a working definition of *case management* and sets out short-term and long-term case management goals. It describes the varied applications of the term and the activities that case managers perform.

Working Definition of Case Management

To be useful, a definition of case management must be both specific and flexible. Although each program needs to develop its own definition, three concepts are essential to a working definition:

1. *It must be comprehensive* for overseeing a patient's entire episode of illness, regardless of the pay class or location in which the service is provided
2. *It must be organized around a system* of interdisciplinary services and resources needed to provide high-quality care in the most cost-effective way
3. *It must be coordinated via clinical and financial management of care* by coordinators, not direct care givers, who have a financial incentive to manage risk and maximize the quality of care.

Each of these concepts is detailed in the following subsections.

Comprehensive System for Entire Episode of Illness

Most so-called case management programs deal with separate components of care, not the continuum of patient care. For example, hospital-initiated case management programs usually deal with the inpatient component, leaving the events that gave rise to the hospitalization and the issues surrounding post-discharge to somebody else or, worse yet, to nobody else.

By design, some case management programs deal with a partial compo-nent of care. Obstetrical case managers, for example, generally deal with new mothers but not with medical problems unrelated to childbirth. Thus, if the new mother develops a cardiac problem, the obstetrical case manager may not be involved in the case. Also by design, some case managers focus on a particular pay class—for example, Medicaid clients—and if the patient is no longer eligible for Medicaid, the case manager's responsibility may ter-minate. Finally, case managers may deal with a subset of "high-risk" patients—regardless of how the term is defined—only for as long as specific criteria are met.

How far can and should case management extend? The most progressive case management programs focus on the patient, *wherever* he or she receives care; they also deal with the patient and family *prior to and after* initiation of the episode of care that warranted the involvement of a case manager. Progressive case management is ongoing—that is, in periods of health as well as sickness—although the levels of care intensity differ depending on need. Some HMOs and some employers, particularly those that are self-insured, have taken this approach.

Two current health care trends, the shift of financial risk from payers to providers and the integration of payers and providers into single systems, will change the rules. Case management in the future is more likely to be compre-hensive than limited in scope.

Systematic Organization of Services and Resources

Historically, the provision of health care has been a segmented series of activi-ties. In response to a fragmented reimbursement system, different provider organi-zations and different departments may be involved in the provision of services for patients—but without coordination of their activities. In most places patient records are fragmented, with separate information systems existing for each insti-tution or provider of care. Systems for measuring costs and outcome—if they exist at all—are primitive and narrowly focused; as a result, it is difficult to know for a given patient receiving care in several locations what the outcome and cost of care were.

Case management can cross provider lines and coordinate care rendered in multiple locations. It also can monitor quality and cost across a continuum of care, helping providers deal with the shifting of financial risk. If patient-focused computerized patient records are available, the patient data base will be more comprehensive than is currently the norm, and case managers thus will have access to data from providers in different sites of care that will enable them to manage the process even more effectively.

Coordinated Clinical and Financial Management of Care

The concept of a "care manager" who can deal with clinical, psychosocial, and financial issues but does not provide care, is an essential component of case management. The coordinator can follow the patient and his or her family and can simultaneously deal with a variety of issues both within and outside the walls of the delivery site.

Case managers in a coordinator role can be valuable resources who are aware of, and have access to, a variety of options for care. They can encourage the use of tools such as clinical paths to help appropriate clinicians deliver care efficiently. They can use outcome data to assess the effectiveness of the delivery process. Because they do not have the responsibility for providing direct care, they can spend time developing relationships and networks. Armed with a vast knowledge of resources, they also can be effective patient advocates.

Goals of Case Management

The development of a case management program requires clarity of purpose. Following are suggestions for primary, secondary, and long-term goals:

- *Primary goal:* To deliver high-quality patient care in the most cost-effective way by managing human and material resources
- *Secondary goals:* To manage the delivery of care within a given time frame; to decrease length of stay for inpatient care; to ensure appropriate utilization of services and resources; to improve continuity of care; to standardize the care delivered for a given diagnosis; to improve patient outcomes from a given episode of care
- *Long-term goal:* Beyond a specific episode of care, to improve overall patient health and well-being with a view of preventing recurrence of illness and the need for health services.

Common Applications of the Term *Case Management*

Although many professionals and organizations claim to do case management, there is no "pure" approach. Most case management programs are qualified by either the target population that they serve (for example, HMO enrollees, home care clients) or by the professionals who perform the job (for example, nurse case managers). Some of the most common applications of the term are:

- Nursing case management
- Product-line or service-line case management

- Geriatric or Medicare case management
- Mental health and substance abuse case management
- Catastrophic case management (for example, for trauma or AIDS patients)
- Home care case management
- HMO (and other health plan) case management
- Employer case management, including workers' compensation
- Medicaid case management

These applications, discussed in the following subsections, have many common features, but they differ with respect to boundaries of responsibility; scope of authority; direct care giver/coordinator of care; use of tools for measurement; and required education and experience. There is no perfect definition—the program model should be developed to achieve the goals agreed on.

Nursing Case Management

The nursing profession has recognized case management as important to both patient care and professional development. The American Nurses Association (ANA 1988) suggests that nurses can perform the role of case manager in three ways: (1) as primary nurses who formally have been given the responsibility for case management; (2) as direct care givers who have no formal responsibility for case management but are interested and become involved as time allows; and (3) as case managers with responsibility for coordination but not direct provision of care.

The work done by Karen Zander and colleagues at New England Medical Center (NEMC) in Boston is an example of primary nurses performing the case management role. Etheredge's book *Collaborative Care: Nursing Case Management* provides a detailed description of the original NEMC efforts (Etheredge 1989):

> In case management, the target of change is the role of the nurse. The change includes accountability for outcomes throughout the episode of illness as well as responsibility for length of stay and the effective use of resources. Case managers are accountable for working with the physician to develop the expected patterns of care by case type and for reviewing those patterns on a regular basis to ensure that they are accurately reflected in case management plans and critical paths. This process establishes the standards of care for the focus case types. . . . the case managers also identify, analyze, and take corrective action for the patterns of variance that emerge within their entire caseload over the entire episode of illness.

Zander's forthcoming book on collaborative care, *Managing Outcomes through Collaborative Care: The Application of Care Mapping and Case Management*, will provide information on the transformation of the nurse case manager model to a multidisciplinary approach.

The second type of nursing case manager model, where interested individuals assume an informal case management role, has often developed into a more formal program. Chapter 9 focusing on Lutheran General Hospital in Park Ridge, Illinois, illustrates the third nursing case management model, in which the case managers are coordinators, not direct care givers.

Nurse case management at St. Mary's Carondelet Hospital and Health Center in Tucson, Arizona, goes beyond the three-part nursing role suggested by the ANA. The Carondelet nursing network involves nurse case managers as both coordinators/brokers *and* as direct care givers in the hospital and in ambulatory and community settings. They have direct and ongoing contact with clients, families, and available resources (Michaels 1994). A detailed description of this unique nurse case management model is presented in chapter 7.

Product-Line or Service-Line Case Management

In product-line or service-line case management programs, the case manager coordinates multidisciplinary services. The model is common in tertiary facilities. For example, the Baptist Memorial Hospital in Memphis, Tennessee, a large tertiary provider (well known as the place where Elvis Presley was pronounced dead on arrival), is renowned for its product-line case management (Southwick 1993; Duncan and Patterson 1993).

Based on the success of a pilot case management program for cardiovascular services, the hospital has converted all of its service lines to a case management system. For each service line (that is, women's health, children's health, neurology/orthopedics, general medicine, surgery, behavioral health, and rehabilitative services), all inpatients have a case manager and a care team. Customized critical paths are used to guide the delivery of care. The overall approach has resulted in significant reductions in length of stay and charges.

Stanford University Hospital in Stanford, California, has had similar success with its service-line case management program (*Hospital Case Management* 1993; Day 1994). In 1989, the 660-bed hospital was in financial difficulty. A multidisciplinary administrative-level task force identified case management as an important survival strategy in a managed care marketplace.

Case management at Stanford began as a pilot program in two areas where physicians had expressed interest in the new approach, urology and oncology. Within months the program had made a significant impact on the bottom line and on patient, family, and staff satisfaction. Case management therefore was extended to cover all patients admitted to the hospital.

The care delivered at Stanford is complex, and the hospital decided to use nurses with clinical expertise as case managers. Existing staff had the opportunity to apply for the job, and, given the clinical strength of a number of nurses, internal candidates qualified for the case manager positions.

Stanford's case managers are not direct care givers; rather, they coordinate the delivery of care and are responsible for discharge planning, utilization review, and, with the nurse managers, the development of clinical paths. Case managers follow patients as they move throughout the hospital, unless the patient's condition requires a shift to another service (and to another case manager). An effective component of the program is the pairing of each case manager with a social worker. As a multidisciplinary team, the case manager and social worker deal with both clinical problems and issues related to insurance coverage. Following discharge, the team remains in contact with patient and family.

Some of the factors that contributed to the success of Stanford's pilot programs and to its subsequent ability to extend case management beyond urology and oncology were the skill level of the clinical nurses, the case manager/social service team concept, and the decision not to use clinical paths at the start. By the time the organization introduced the clinical path concept, case management had already been accepted. (Figure 3-1 contains examples of clinical paths and other tools that case managers can use, and figure 3-2 is a sample clinical path.)

The reporting relationship of the case management program was also important. The director of utilization management and social work is also in charge of the case managers and reports directly to the associate director of patient care services. The direct report to patient care services has helped to strengthen the day-to-day relationship between the case managers and nurses who render direct care.

Future plans call for the introduction of an automated information system that will interface with the hospital system. Case managers will use laptop computers to enter and access patient information. (Note: In the fall of 1994, Stanford reorganized case management into a new quality support department reporting directly to the chief medical officer. The change was made to better integrate many activities that had previously been separate: precertification, risk management, accreditation, and outcomes management [Day 1994].)

Although product-line case management has produced good results, especially in tertiary facilities, it has one major disadvantage—application to a patient who reenters the health care system for a reason unrelated to the product line. Because of this shortcoming, in nontertiary settings providers may prefer a one-on-one relationship between case manager and patient that remains in place over time, regardless of the specific health care service needed.

Geriatric or Medicare Case Management

Geriatric patients, of course, are a unique population whose psychosocial or economic circumstances may influence their medical needs in hidden as well as obvious ways. To assist hospitals in dealing with high-risk, high-cost Medicare patients, United Healthcare Corporation in Minneapolis, Minnesota, developed a geriatric case management program that hospitals can purchase in order to manage a subset of Medicare patients (*Hospital Peer Review* 1990). The outside case management program coordinates closely with the activities performed by the client hospital's own staff.

Another example of geriatric case management is the program for a multi-level retirement community that is managed by the University of Washington School of Nursing in partnership with a private corporation (Young and Haight 1993). The program is institution-focused and is geared toward moving residents appropriately between different levels of care (that is, independent living, assisted living, and skilled nursing) as the need arises. The case management services are available to all residents but are most important for those unable to negotiate their own way through the system.

Mental Health and Substance Abuse Case Management

The many examples of case management for mental health and substance abuse patients suggest both widespread use of the concept. They also suggest some of the difficulties inherent in measuring outcome in terms of cost efficiency or quality of life.

Four common case management programs for mental health patients are expanded broker, personal strength, rehabilitation, and full-support (Clark and Fox 1993). The four variations are described following:

- *Expanded broker case managers* assess client needs and develop linkages to appropriate services, but they do not provide care.
- *Personal strength case managers* match client strengths with those situations most likely to facilitate good achievement.
- *Rehabilitation case managers* focus on client deficits and on the skills needed to overcome them.
- *Full-support case managers* are both direct care givers and coordinator/brokers for care that they do not provide themselves.

For all of these models, an important determinant of the impact of case management is who makes the decision, the client or the case manager. There may be more of a client-controlled chain of events than there is in nonmental health/substance abuse case management, where patients are more likely to comply with a recommended course of action.

In a comprehensive overview of eight studies of case management programs for patients with severe and chronic mental illness, Rubin notes that in spite of the general consensus that case management does slow down the "revolving door" of service delivery, empirical evidence on the outcome is questionable (Rubin 1992). A major difficulty is ability to isolate the impact of the case management function from that of the total package of care provided. Another common problem is the obstacle the case manager encounters when the recommended services are not available or reimbursable.

For substance abuse patients, the case management concept often involves treating more than the substance abuse problem (Woodward, no date available). For example, case managers might deal with issues related to pregnancy, homelessness, poverty, unemployment, and problems other than the alcohol or drug abuse.

Catastrophic Case Management

Patients with AIDS, trauma, and other multiple medical and nonmedical needs that inevitably cross service delivery lines are logical targets for the case management approach (Simmons 1992). Trauma patients, for example, may arrive by helicopter or ambulance, enter into the health care system through the emergency department, and then require a variety of services and postdischarge care. Sharp HealthCare in San Diego has designated a trauma case manager (TCM) to coordinate care, and its program is described in detail in chapter 8.

Community Medical Alliance (CMA) in Boston has developed a case management approach for AIDS patients and for patients with multiple handicaps who qualify for personal care attendants. Over a four-year period, CMA has provided and/or coordinated services for 600 people, including 15 percent of all AIDS patients and 50 percent of all severely handicapped patients in greater Boston (Rosenbloom 1994).

Referral to CMA is made by a provider or friend. Patients who qualify on a clinical basis enroll with CMA with the permission of the insurance carrier. Then CMA assumes responsibility for both the direct care and coordination of all services, regardless of setting. Emphasis is on noninstitutional care, and patients receive most of their care in the home or other ambulatory setting.

CMA has its own provider network of medical groups, independent medical contractors, and ancillary services. The key care givers are primary care physicians and nurse practitioners. Particularly the nurse practitioners develop close relationships with patients, families, and support groups and act as the "case managers."

Case management and direct care from CMA is patient-focused and is available 24 hours a day, seven days a week. The access to care and to coordination of care distinguishes CMA from health care organizations/institutions that are inflexible in meeting patient or family needs. Other distinguishing characteristics of the CMA case management program are the importance of the personal relationship between patients/families and clinicians, and the use of the team concept.

A number of tools are available to assist with AIDS case management. The American Medical Association (AMA) and the Agency for Health Care Policy and Research (AHCPR) both have guidelines for managing the care of HIV-infected persons (*Case Management Advisor* 1994b). To help providers manage complicated cases, Automated Case Management Systems, Inc., of Studio City, California, has developed software for use by social service agencies caring for AIDS patients (Swoben 1993).

Home Care Case Management

The idea of case management in the home setting is not new. Prior to the growth of technology and the provision of care in institutional settings, patients received most of their care at home. Physicians, nurses, and, ultimately, organized home health and visiting nurse organizations provided case management, although they may not have used that term. Not all family members worked, so that professional care givers often had the added benefit of lay assistance.

Today's home care professionals who provide case management have different challenges from those that confront case managers in other settings. In all likelihood, the former will be called on to deal with issues related to transportation, acquisition and delivery of supplies and equipment, safety, provision of education and support to care givers, and varying reimbursement policies (Donovan 1993). As prospective payment, capitation arrangements, and plan-specific policies promote earlier discharge from institutional settings, patients will continue to arrive home "sooner and sicker," and they and their families will need a great deal of help in dealing with problems formerly handled by physicians and nurses in the inpatient setting.

HMO Case Management

Given the risk basis of the HMO concept and the nature of capitation, HMOs may use case management to manage their enrollee populations. Hinitz-Satterfield, Miller, and Hagan, for example, distinguish the broad role of the HMO nursing case manager (NCM) from the more limited role of the utilization case manager.

> The NCM "literally follows as the patient moves along a broad continuum of services and sites of care, acting to connect and coordinate separate events into a unity of adaptation and health maintenance. This therapeutic whole is much greater than the mere summing of well-orchestrated parts. Although the NCM is responsible for ensuring that referrals are orderly and transitions are smooth, the true professional meaning and worth of the role are expressed in the ability to preserve and promote healthy outcomes during periods of transition and risk" (Hinitz-Satterfield, Miller, and Hagan 1993).

At least three characteristics of HMO case management programs distinguish them from provider-based programs. First, some HMO programs are limited to covered beneficiaries, not to other family members who may have different health insurance coverage but may be key to the management of the total case. Second, some HMOs focus case management on chart review and ignore or minimize personal interaction with patient and family. Finally, in many instances the health plan and providers may have contractual relationships but not be integrated formally into the system; the HMO and provider may each have their own case managers. As a result, from a patient/family viewpoint, there may be confusion over the duplicative roles of the HMO-based and provider-based staff.

One example of an HMO with a case management component is the Phoenix Health Plan (PHP) in Arizona (Munir 1994). The PHP is owned by PMH Health Resources, Inc., and is part of a system that includes Phoenix Memorial Hospital, three regional campuses, a multisite network of family health and occupational medicine centers, a freestanding urgent care center, and a 200-physician, physician–hospital organization.

The plan began in 1984, and within 10 years its enrollment included more than 30,000 Medicaid recipients in three categories: children age 0 to 21, pregnant women, and other adults who qualify for assistance because of disability or indigence. By 1994, the plan was preparing for an accreditation review by the National Committee for Quality Assurance.

Initially, PHP offered case management for "catastrophic" cases, that is, those enrollees whose diagnosis or level of claims paid might benefit from extra coordination of patient care. Plan staff quickly realized that many of the nurses with prior experience in home health care, infusion therapy, and medical/surgical care could provide special coordinating services for enrollees who did not require extensive services—thus, the "case management" function was born.

Also by 1994, PHP had five case managers who report to the utilization management coordinator and who work closely with four concurrent review nurses. The case managers specialize by demographic subset; for example, adult, pediatrics, or obstetrics. Particularly those case managers who specialize in adult care deal with nonmedical needs such as transportation, noncompliance with physician orders, or medication requirements.

Not all enrollees have case managers, but the case managers do review the full records of all enrollees who are admitted as inpatients to determine whether a case manager should be assigned. The case managers also act as resources for the primary care physicians, suggesting alternative care that may enable patients to receive care outside the hospital setting and circumvent unnecessary admission.

Within a systems context, the PHP case managers work closely with hospital patient care coordinators so that the transition from inpatient to outpatient environment is smooth. The patient care coordinators focus on what happens to patients within the walls of the hospital during an inpatient stay, and, if appropriate, the case managers take over following discharge.

The PHP case managers differ from the case managers at other health plans in two important ways: location of their operational base, and clinical experience. As resources and not direct care givers, they are located in the health plan office. They attend selected discharge planning and patient care conferences whenever they can be helpful in facilitating these meetings, but they use the health plan office as their geographic base to increase access for physicians, office staff, and other care givers. The approach that has cut down on telephone tag. In other plans, case managers spend more time in the field and have more direct interaction with patients, families, and care givers.

The PHP case managers, hired from outside the plan, are experienced nurse clinicians with backgrounds in home health care and home infusion services. Other plans and health care organizations retrain existing staff for the case management position, but PHP felt that experience in the nonacute setting was a particularly valuable asset.

Employer Case Management

In focusing on strategies to encourage wellness and reduce the cost of providing health care, employers have taken some creative approaches toward case management. To some of the more active employers, provider-based case management is equivalent to the fox guarding the chicken coop, and they are adamant about the need for their own involvement.

The use of case management for workers' compensation cases is fairly common, and some employers recognize significant cost savings by buying workers' compensation and employee health insurance from the same managed care carrier (Health Care Advisory Board 1994). For example, in Massachusetts, employers can purchase an HMO or a PPO product plus "Managed Comp" from the Tufts Associated Health Plan, using the same provider network for both. The strategy shifts workers' compensation out of the fee-for-service arena and discourages employees from "double-dipping," that is, seeking care under both types of coverage.

Some employers have developed their own elaborate systems to manage employee health and wellness. An example is Parker-Hannifin, a Cleveland-based Fortune 200 producer of manufacturing components and motion control systems, with 20,000 employees (Roos, Munsell, and Blake 1993). The company's "self-management" program features *health care coordinators*, registered nurses (RNs) and support staff employed by the company to assist all employees and their dependents in managing both health and illness.

The Parker-Hannifin health care coordinators are *resources*, not providers, who guide enrollees through four possible phases of health and illness: prevention and wellness promotion; early assistance with employee health care needs; back-to-work assistance (for example, worker's compensation, disability, and employee assistance programs [EAPs]); and patient care management (for example, preadmission review, hospital utilization review, case management, and coordination at all levels). The self-management program emphasis is on prevention and wellness, and its goal is to keep employees healthy.

General Electric (GE) Aircraft Engines in Lynn, Massachusetts, is another example of employer management of employees' health and wellness. Although a formal case management program does not link the components together, GE's programs do cover the broad spectrum of needs.

Using a derivative of the SF-36 health status questionnaire developed at the Rand Corporation, GE annually assesses employees' functional health status. The questionnaires take into account work, social life, and leisure-time activities. Information from the surveys enables the company to focus its wellness programs and to identify areas for secondary prevention. For example, primary care prevention (that is, keeping the well healthy) is handled through on-site health and fitness center programs related to exercise, nutrition, stress, and lifestyle management and through plantwide programs for injury prevention and ergonomics. Secondary prevention, directed toward groups at risk for a particular disease or condition, include examples such as early detection programs for breast health, high blood pressure and cholesterol monitoring, and smoking cessation. Tertiary prevention strategies deal with employees who already have been ill and are identified as being at high risk. Finally, the Convalescence Assistance for Recovering Employees (CARE) program provides on-site medical center support to employees who have been out of work because of illness or injury (Galvin 1993).

Other employers believe that case management can best be done by an outside company, rather than by the employer or insurance carrier. Marriott Corporation in Bethesda, Maryland, and Ciba-Geigy Corporation are two such examples.

One company that works with many large employers to manage their health care costs is the Franklin Health Group (FHG) in Ramsey, New Jersey. The FGH health care cost-management methodology was developed to deal with a fact that many employers forget—that a small percentage of covered beneficiaries accounts for a large share of health care costs (Levy and Hines 1994).

Following a cost analysis and identification of "manageable cost areas," a physician-led FHG team looks at patient diagnoses and conditions and works with employees, family members, and other parties (for example, insurance carriers) to see if intervention—and perhaps alternative treatment plans—will produce more satisfactory results. Employee participation is voluntary, and the patient acceptance rate has been 90 percent.

Medicaid Case Management

Because Medicaid clients may have social, economic, and nonmedical needs that have impact on their ability to access and use medical care, it is no surprise that there are Medicaid-specific case management programs. In fact, since Congress authorized optional case management services under Medicaid in 1981, at least 40 states have developed programs (*Case Management Advisor* 1994a).

For example, in 1992 the Commonwealth of Massachusetts implemented an innovative Medicaid managed care program for several large categories of recipients. The key program feature was the primary care clinician (PCC) concept, and participants were expected to select a PCC from a list of participating fee-for-service physicians. Recipients also had the option to select a managed care plan.

Two years after the inception of managed Medicaid, the Medical Assistance Division of the Massachusetts Department of Public Welfare issued a Request for Proposal for case management for this population. The proposed program scope included medical care coordination, recipient support, and administrative support (Massachusetts Department of Public Welfare 1993).

The Activities of Case Management

Although applications of the case management concept vary, all case managers must perform five basic tasks. These tasks—assessment, planning, intervention, monitoring, and evaluation (Redford 1992)—are discussed in more detail in the following subsections.

Assessment

All case managers must obtain factual information about the patient and family. A combination of standardized and problem-focused assessment factors is commonly used. The scope of the assessment is broad, covering personal and environmental factors as well as medical information. A good example of information that case managers obtain in the assessment phase is the determination of whether the patient lives alone. A patient who lives alone may have very supportive family members who can assist in providing care, whereas a married patient living with a spouse dealing with his or her own health problems may need more assistance.

Planning

The plan that emerges from the needs assessment becomes the care road map. The plan should be multidisciplinary and include medical and nonmedical care and services that will be provided by physicians, nurses, other professional care givers, and supporting family and friends. Furthermore, it should contain goals stated in terms of clinically desirable and financially feasible outcomes. A clinical map—that is, a "written process standard that reflects a multidisciplinary approach to cost-effective, quality patient care"—is the generic term applied to such a plan (Riegel and others 1993).

Intervention

Implementation of a case management plan is a challenging process. A comprehensive plan will cover a continuum of care including, but not limited to, medical care. To facilitate intervention (direct and indirect), case managers need a vast knowledge of available resources and the ability to tactfully orchestrate the delicate process of negotiation among patient/client, family, support system, and available resources. For example, in families where an elderly parent's post-discharge care is dependent on siblings' cooperation, a case manager may have to intervene to ease negative family dynamics.

Monitoring

There are formal and informal ways to make sure that the case management plan that has been laid out is followed, and that variance is measured. By focusing on the variance, providers can identify the source of a problem and take appropriate steps for correction. The clinical map (mentioned under the section on planning and other tools described in figure 3-1) may offer sophisticated methods for measuring variance from expected clinician performance and patient outcome.

Evaluation

Case management is not a static process, and its assessment and evaluation need to reinforce the importance of flexibility. Organizations most successful in their evaluations have looked at program structure and process on a continuous basis and have not presumed that the original program design would remain appropriate over time. As integrated systems evolve, ongoing reassessment is particularly important.

References and Bibliography

American Nurses Association. *Case Management: A Challenge for Nurses.* Kansas City, MO: ANA, 1988.

Case Management Advisor 5(3):29, Mar. 1994a. (Newsletter published by American Health Consultants, Inc., Atlanta, GA.)

Case Management Advisor 5(4):51–53, Apr. 1994b. (Newsletter published by American Health Consultants, Inc., Atlanta, GA.)

Clark, R. E., and Fox, T. S. A framework for evaluating the economic impact of case management. *Hospital and Community Psychiatry* 44(5):469–73, 1993.

Day, C. Telephone interviews with director of social services and utilization management, Stanford University Hospital, Stanford, CA, Apr. 18, 25, and Sept. 26, 1994.

Donovan, M. R. Case management as a foundation for home care. In: D. Lerman and E. B. Linne, editors. *Hospital Home Care.* Chicago: American Hospital Publishing, Inc., 1993.

Duncan, K., and Patterson, J. Enhancing outcomes with case management. *The Journal of Cardiovascular Management* 4(3):33–39, May–June 1993.

Etheredge, M. L. S., editor. *Collaborative Care: Nursing Case Management.* Chicago: American Hospital Publishing, Inc., 1989, p. 11.

Galvin, R. S. Interviews with manager of health care management and medical services, General Electric Aircraft Engines, Lynn, MA, Nov. and Dec. 1993, and May 1994.

The Health Care Advisory Board. *Combining Workers' Compensation, Employee Health Benefits Aids Cost Containment.* Washington, DC: HCAB, Feb. 9, 1994.

Hinitz-Satterfield, P., Miller, E. H., and Hagan, E. P. Managing nursing care: promises and pitfalls. Chapter 6 in *Utilization and Case Management in an HMO.* Series on Nursing Administration 5, 1993, pp. 83–99.

Hospital Peer Review. Geriatric care managers: intruders or saviors? *Hospital Peer Review* 15(3):44–47, Mar. 9, 1990.

Is case management the answer to coping with managed care? *Hospital Case Management* 1(6):104–8, 111, June 1993.

Levy, D., and Hines, D. J. Telephone interviews with the Franklin Health Group, Apr. 13, 26, 1994.

Massachusetts Department of Public Welfare. *Request for Proposal for Case Management Program for Medicaid Recipients.* July 7, 1993.

Michaels, C. Telephone interview with professional nurse case manager and clinical director of research, Carondelet St. Mary's Hospital and Health System, Apr. 8, 1994.

Munir, N. Telephone interview with medical director, Phoenix Health Plan, Mar. 11, 1994.

Redford, L. J. Case management, the wave of the future. *Journal of Case Management* 1(1):5–8, Spring 1992.

Riegel, B., Tomlinson, C., Weiss, M., Saks, N., Glancy, M., and Hanley, P. *Sharp HealthCare Manual for Clinical Mapping.* San Diego, CA: Sharp HealthCare, Nov. 1993.

Roos, T. S., Munsell, J. M., and Blake, W. D. Parker-Hannifin's health benefits program: self-management. *Managed Care Quarterly* 1(4):1–11, 1993.

Rosenbloom, D. L. Interview with Community Medical Alliance, Boston, MA, May 2, 1994.

Rubin, A. Is case management effective for people with serious mental illness? A research review. *Health and Social Work* 17(2):138–50, May 1992.

Simmons, F. M. Developing the trauma nurse case manager role. *Dimension of Critical Care Nursing* 11(3):164–70, May–June 1992.

Southwick, K. Memphis' huge Baptist Memorial fast-tracks institution-wide case management for quality and efficiency gains. *Strategies for Healthcare Excellence* 6(11):1-8, Nov. 1993.

Swoben, J. M-based case management system helps coordinate care for AIDS patients. *Computers in Health Care M Technology, Special Edition* June 1993, pp. 12-13.

Travis, M. and Gwordz, D. T. Nursing case management for patients with TURP. *Urologic Nursing* 13(2):48-54, June 1993.

Woodward, A. *Managed Care and Case Management of Substance Abuse Treatment.* Rockville, MD: National Institute of Drug Abuse, pp. 34-53. (No date available.)

Young, H. M. and Haight, K. Case management in a retirement community. *Nursing Administration Quarterly* 17(3):34-8, Spring 1993.

Zander, K. *Managing Outcomes through Collaborative Care: The Application of Care Mapping and Case Management.* Chicago: American Hospital Publishing, 1995.

Chapter Two

Why Is Case Management Necessary?

Health care reform is the number-one item on executive, legislative, organizational, and corporate agendas. Major changes in health care financing and delivery already have occurred at the state and community levels.

As they rethink their approaches to patient care, providers need a good grasp of the important components of the "new" health care. In keeping with the principles of total quality management, senior managers must also be able to explain the key principles of these components to all levels of the organization.

This chapter answers the question "Why is case management necessary?" It describes the current environment and explains important concepts (managed care, American Hospital Association community care networks,* and integrated financing and delivery systems). The chapter also discusses the roles that key players (that is, the public policy makers, public and private payers, and health plans) already have assumed and examines the pressure for provider accountability. Finally, the chapter describes the new role for providers.

Important Concepts

This section lays out major concepts relevant to the new health care climate. These include managed care responsibility shared among providers, consumers, and payers; AHA's community care networks based on collaboration and accountability; and integrated financing and delivery systems.

What Is Managed Care?

Experts predict that the country is quickly moving toward a scenario where most of the population covered by health insurance will be in managed care. The experts, however, do not agree on the meaning of the term.

---

*Community Care Network, Inc., uses the name Community Care Network as its service mark and reserves all rights.

Managed care refers to "a wide range of health care delivery and payment strategies designed to hold down costs while assuring quality of care" (Lewin-VHI 1993). Managed care includes types of insurance plans (for example, traditional indemnity, HMO, PPO, and so on), and it includes strategies (for example, selective contracting or utilization management) that target one or more of the components of health spending, such as utilization, price, and intensity of care. As it evolves, managed care implies shared obligations and responsibilities by providers, consumers, and payers.

Providers

Historically providers have assumed that they know what is best for their patients, and that external attempts by insurance companies and reviewers to micromanage patient care is an inappropriate intrusion. As financial risk shifts from payers to providers, however, providers are learning to understand that they themselves are responsible for both the provision and management of care. They need internally driven, not externally set, standards for care that demonstrate high-quality and cost-effective delivery.

Consumers

Given the way in which the health care system currently is structured, consumers—who may at some time become patients—have applied a double standard in making their purchasing decisions. For non–health care items they can be smart shoppers both in terms of their initial purchase and in product maintenance. They may, for example, use consumer publications to guide their purchase of a car, and they are likely to abide by recommended schedules for routine maintenance, repair, and inspection.

The average consumer's approach to purchasing health care services, however, has not demonstrated smart shopping; and, in view of the traditional health insurance mechanism, consumers in general have been less than responsible. Under the future managed care scenario, they will have to buy smarter and assume more responsibility for their own health as well as for their use of the health care system during an illness episode.

Payers

Traditionally perceived by providers and consumers as the bad guys who manage care by limiting benefit coverage or denying payment, payers will join with providers to emphasize both wellness and a different approach to the treatment of illness. They will lay out expectations for providers and demand quality care at a price they can afford.

American Hospital Association Community Care Networks

The vision for reform set forth by the AHA focuses on the community care network (AHA 1993). Various other organizations have proposed similar structures using different terminology. Key to the concept is the idea that collaboration will improve a community's health status through the provision of a seamless continuum of services by health care providers operating within a fixed budget. Accountability is to the community.

As envisioned by AHA, the community care network concept encompasses four goals:

1. Refocusing attention on patients and communities
2. Emphasizing prevention as a means to minimize illness and disability
3. Improving the system's user friendliness
4. Realigning the incentives that have impact on behavior with regard to the use of health care resources

Within this broad framework, each community network is expected to be unique, but all networks will have these common characteristics:

- *Focus on community health:* Networks would provide services not only to enrolled populations, but would be responsible for reaching out to the community-at-large to assess health needs and, with other organizations, to develop programs to meet those needs.
- *Seamless continuum of care:* Networks would address the fragmented nature of existing delivery systems by creating user-friendly networks and by making sure that the different components were coordinated.
- *Management within fixed resources:* The networks would receive risk-adjusted capitated payments to provide care for the enrolled population.
- *Community accountability:* Networks would be expected to demonstrate accountability to patients and the public; measures of quality and performance would provide appropriate feedback; and opportunity for public representation in network governance would be available.

To make the notion of responsibility for the care of a given community work, techniques such as case management can effectively bring together disparate resources and levels of care.

Integrated Financing and Delivery Systems

Integrated financing and delivery systems is the phrase used to describe the future configuration of health care. As described by The Advisory Board (The Advisory

Board 1993a, 1993b), some of the important features of these systems will be as follows:

- *Vertical integration of services,* where different levels of care (for example, primary and specialist, acute, subacute, long-term, ambulatory, and home-based) will be linked together in a seamless *continuum,* and patients who access care will move smoothly among the different components.
- *Payment by capitation,* where the unit of value is cost per member per month. Health care systems that include both providers and payers will be financially at risk and responsible for a specific defined population assigned to them. Managing within budget will mean keeping that assigned population as healthy as possible, so that when individuals do get sick there will be money to pay for the care needed.
- *Low-cost/high-quality services* that are priced below market value and that satisfy purchasers' need for "value-added services."
- *Rationing of resources* in several ways: Primary care physicians will have more formal responsibility for coordinating patient care and will become very active "gatekeepers" who direct their patients toward specialty and institutional care. Benefit coverage may be redefined; in some cases it will extend coverage, but in other cases limit it.

Integrated financing and delivery systems have already been developed in California, Minnesota, and other states (Grant 1993; Minnesota's Integrated Service Networks 1993). The work done by Stephen Shortell at Northwestern University in Evanston, Illinois, provides excellent information on their structure, operations, and four-stage development (Shortell 1993).

In general, systems formed for market-related reasons rather than in response to the needs of specific immigrant and/or religious groups or for capital formation are well positioned to meet the needs of the future (Jones and Mayerhofer 1994). Moreover—and much to the dismay of many hospital CEOs—hospitals are not necessarily the best starting points for systems formation (Morrison 1994).

Regardless of the reasons they form, however, systems incorporate care delivered at multiple levels and in all likelihood, at multiple locations. Case management can "glue" the parts together.

Transitional Strategies

In most regions of the country, providers and payers are not yet organized into integrated financing and delivery systems, and some may never get there at all, making life complicated for health policy makers (Jones and Mayerhofer 1994). Most places are in a transitional stage; and in preparation for the ultimate goal that they see before them, they are experimenting with a variety of transitional strategies including, but not limited to, the following (The Advisory Board 1993b):

- Management service bureaus (MSBs)
- Group practice without walls
- Open or closed physician–hospital associations (PHOs)
- Comprehensive management service organizations (CMSOs)
- Foundation model
- Staff model
- Equity model

Regardless of where providers currently are in systems development, success will depend on the capability to assume financial risk and to coordinate the clinical delivery of care (Conrad 1993). Case management can enhance that capability.

Key Players in the Health Care Scenario

Many key players will determine the future of health care in the United States. They are public policy makers, public payers, private payers, and providers themselves. The following discussions describe what roles each might play and the influence they might exert.

Federal Government

As public policy on a national health program evolves, a number of key issues repeatedly arise. Among them are universal access, economic discipline, financing, and administration, employer responsibility, and regulatory excess. In addition, the balance between national and state roles continues to be an important and delicate issue. Each of these themes is described in the following list:

1. *Universal access and standardized coverage:* Health care in the United States is significantly tied to employment and historically has not been uniformly available to all citizens. Comprehensive national health reform would need to address universal access to a federally defined standard benefit package.
2. *Economic discipline:* There is wide disparity in the method by which U.S. citizens purchase health insurance. Employment status, employer size, and preexisting health conditions all affect the availability and price of care. Purchasing coalitions and other buyer techniques could address some of the inequities.
3. *Financing:* Any expanded access to health care will be costly. Potential funding sources are increased employer obligations, reductions in Medicare and Medicaid payments to providers, and/or an increase in "sin taxes."
4. *Administration:* If national health care reform were to weather the political process, a new regulatory body might be needed to set standards and oversee the establishment and operation of the new system. Among the most

important of a new board/agency's responsibilities would be the establishment and maintenance of a national quality management program.

State-Level Activities

At the state level, there have been two approaches to the health care dilemma.
Some states have clearly indicated that they will make no changes in health
care unless they are required to do so. Other states already have taken aggres-
sive steps to make changes in health care financing and/or delivery.

Although health care providers need to pay closest attention to efforts going
on in their particular states, they can broaden their perspective by understanding
major initiatives in other parts of the country. By doing so, they will have a
realistic context into which they can place the case management programs they
develop.

As described by Jesse Helms in testimony before Congress (Helms 1993),
leading states are pursuing three types of strategies:

1. *Strategies for improving financial access* (for example, new tax-financed systems such as payroll, income, provider, and sin taxes; mandates for
   employers, individuals and/or families; subsidies for the uninsured and other
   groups; restructuring of the insurance market through purchasing cooperatives, small group reforms, and so on)
2. *Strategies for controlling costs* (for example, expenditure targets and caps; rate
   setting; managed competition through purchasing cooperatives; and improvements in administrative efficiency [electronic billing, claims processing, and
   remittance, for example])
3. *Strategies for the improvement of health delivery systems* (for example, develop-
   ment/encouragement of integrated service networks and improvements in
   access for underserved populations by primary care initiatives)

Public and Private Payers

Faced with dramatic increases in the cost of health insurance, many public
and private payers have already made changes in their health care benefit programs. Their activities include:

- *Willingness to reduce the range of choices:* Once fearful of reducing employee
  choice of health care, especially for large numbers of employees, employers
  have changed their approach. Looking for long-term, cost-effective solutions
  to rapidly escalating costs, many large companies are casting their lots with
  a single company. Other employers not only are reducing the number of
  available options, but are limiting premium inflation with multiyear agree-
  ments. When employers use such approaches, they may add case management as well to facilitate the changes for their employees and dependents.

- *Methodological evaluation of health insurance options:* Faced with skyrocketing costs, employers have become much more analytical in their scrutiny of different health insurance options. Many have adopted the report card approach to compare health insurance options (Bergman 1994a).
- *Formation of purchasing coalitions:* No longer content to approach health insurance on a company-specific basis, employers in many communities have banded together in purchasing coalitions. Together they have been able to develop and implement standards for quality of care, limit the rate of premium increase, and hold providers more accountable.
- *Increased comfort with employee cost sharing:* Many employers historically have been reluctant to pass on a portion of the cost of health care to their employees. As the cost of care and insurance has risen, however, employee cost sharing has become more prevalent. As employees assume some financial responsibility for health benefits, they are more careful in the insurance plans they select and in the care they access. Thus they will be more cognizant of quality of care and gaps in service delivery, two areas that case management can address.
- *Carve-out products:* As their sophistication in health benefits management has grown, employers have identified high-cost areas, separated them out from their regular health insurance plans, and added special case management programs. Mental health and substance abuse, for example, are often funded and managed in a different way from other services.
- *Direct contracting:* In some (not all) areas of the country, employers have bypassed the insurance companies and contracted directly with providers. Third-party administrators (TPAs) frequently handle the administrative, marketing, and claims payment functions. Strong case management is often put in place to help manage these special programs.

Given all these changes regarding health insurance in both public and private sectors, providers with a case management approach can develop a competitive advantage with health plans, employers and other group purchasers, and consumers.

Health Plans

Health plan initiatives (for example, product diversification, plan consolidation, selective contracting, and risk shifting) are all directed toward controlling cost while maintaining quality. Case management often accompanies new plan strategies.

- *Product diversification:* Hoping to entice employers to select a "replacement" for current multiple options, insurers have diversified their offerings. Many now offer tightly controlled HMO plans, along with less restrictive preferred provider organizations (PPOs) and/or point-of-service (POS) options. As mentioned in chapter 1, some plans are adding a workers' compensation product.

- *Consolidation:* In many parts of the country, health plans have combined their resources. In order to provide a wide array of options within a single plan, staff, group, and IPA model HMO plans may merge formally, or they may prefer a loose affiliation with joint marketing. In a different type of consolidation, plans with circumscribed service areas are forming regional combinations. For example, the Pacific Integrated Healthcare (PIH) regional integrated delivery system announced in spring 1994 would unite Adventist Health System/West with Loma Linda University Medical Center. Loma Linda is the medical affiliate of Friendly Hills HealthCare Network (*Managed Care Week, Integration Trends for Managed Care Plans* 1994).
- *Selective contracting:* To obtain better rates in return for larger volume, many plans are taking a selective rather than an inclusive approach toward hospitals and physicians. Nonetheless, in some states "any willing provider" laws requiring that plans contract with all qualified providers who are willing to accept their payments are thwarting such efforts.
- *Shifting of risk from payers to providers:* Methods of payment for care are shifting rapidly, moving away from those that place the payer at risk (for example, discounted charges and per diems), to those that place providers at risk (for example, per case, global hospital/physician payments, and capitation).

Pressures for Accountability

The pressure on hospital and physician providers to demonstrate accountability for the care they deliver has increased. Although the marketplace may be slow to come forward with financial recognition for quality, even over the long run, health plans, insurers, and employers are improving their capabilities to set quality and utilization standards, and to hold providers accountable (The Advisory Board 1993d).

Among the groups already looking at quality and outcomes information are the Joint Commission for Accreditation of Healthcare Organizations (JCAHO) and the National Committee for Quality Assurance (NCQA) in Washington, D.C. The JCAHO Indicator Monitoring System (IMS), for example, measures both actual clinical care and management of the health care organization (*Joint Commission Perspectives* 1993). Already, some states have developed quality and outcome standards. The Physician Payment Review Commission has done work with physician profiling; that is, the concept of looking at patterns of care, not single episodes, and making comparisons with an established norm (Welch and others 1994).

One of the more interesting frameworks for accountability is the Health Plan Employer Data and Information Set (HEDIS) developed by representatives of employers and health plans, along with NCQA. HEDIS calls for compiling and reporting health plan performance so that purchasers, and eventually consumers, can select plans on the basis of quality of care and value. The plans themselves are expected to use the information to measure and improve their own performance. HEDIS 2.0 defines quality as: access to care, appropriateness, efficacy, technical outcome, and member satisfaction (Business and Health 1993). Case management can facilitate high-quality care as measured by these standards.

Providers in a Changing Environment

Once the hub of patient care activity, hospitals are coming to understand their changing (and diminishing) role in the health care system of the future. Morrison compares the hospitals of the 1990s with the railways of the late nineteenth century. Once "the lifeblood of the American transportation system, . . . the railways faded into bit players in the last century." He predicts that hospitals will face a similar fate in the twentieth century and must examine their future options (Morrison 1994).

Inpatient care is decreasing, causing a shift to ambulatory services and home-based care. Those patients who need to be hospitalized are the very sickest, for whom alternative care is inappropriate. As the inpatient/outpatient balance shifts, many hospitals are looking at *reengineering*, defined by Hammer as "the radical redesign of the critical systems and processes used to produce, deliver, and support patient care in order to achieve dramatic improvements in organizational performance within a short period of time" (Bergman 1994b).

Many communities have witnessed a rash of hospital mergers and consolidations, as well as downsizing and closures. Guided by the AHA community care network effort, hospitals are looking for new relationships among different levels of service, with the recognition that community health information networks will make those linkages work (*Hospitals and Health Networks* 1994).

As their own place in the health care scenario changes, hospitals are linking closely with physicians. In the more advanced systems, hospitals, physicians, and insurers have become true economic partners, with shared risk and responsibility. Less advanced systems (still evident in most of the country), are characterized by physician–hospital organizations (PHOs), management service organizations (MSOs), group practices without walls, and other configurations that are probably transitional.

Like hospitals, physicians understand that change is on the way. In many communities, solo practice is becoming virtually extinct, as physicians move into structures/organizations that are better able to assume and manage risk. In some cases these are single specialty groups; in others they are large multi-specialty groups.

Primary care is in its ascendancy. In the future, patients will be encouraged to seek primary care treatment/coordination for all care. Specialist physicians will see a change in referral patterns, and funding for physician training will be heavily weighted toward primary care.

The method by which health care is purchased is changing dramatically. Hospitals and physicians will become increasingly dependent on health plans that route huge blocks of enrollees toward preferred providers and away from "nonpreferred" providers. The relationship between providers and consumers will become more distant as health plans and purchasing coalitions come between them (The Advisory Board 1993c).

The growth of health care spending will come to a grinding halt. The proposed savings in expenditures as well as methods of payment that shift risk to providers will lower provider revenues. Even the additional dollars gained from increased access to care for those who now lack it will not make up the shortfall (The Advisory Board 1993c).

The bottom line for both hospitals and physicians is that to compete and survive in the current and future environment, they need to learn new techniques for managing a broad spectrum of care. Case management is a logical starting place.

References and Bibliography

The Advisory Board. *Vision of the Future.* Washington, DC: The Advisory Board Company, 1993a.

The Advisory Board. *The Grand Alliance: Vertical Integration Strategies for Physicians and Health Systems.* Washington, DC: The Advisory Board Company, 1993b.

The Advisory Board. *The Year Ahead: Briefing for Hospital Board Members on the President's Plan for Health Reform.* Washington, DC: The Advisory Board Company, 1993c.

The Advisory Board. *Outcomes Strategy, Measurement of Hospital Quality under Reform.* Volume 1. Washington, DC: The Advisory Board Company, 1993d.

American Hospital Association. *Transforming Health Care Delivery: Toward Community Care Networks.* Chicago: American Hospital Association, 1993.

Bergman, R. Making the grade. *Hospitals and Health Networks* 68(1):34–36, Jan. 5, 1994a.

Bergman, R. Reengineering health care. *Hospitals and Health Networks* 68(3):28–36, Feb. 5, 1994b.

Business and Health. HEDIS 2.0: A precursor to national report cards for health plans. *Business and Health* 11(14):14, Dec. 1993.

Conrad, D. A. Coordinating patient care services in regional health systems: the challenge of clinical integration. *Journal of the Foundation of the American College of Healthcare Executives* 38(4):491–507, Winter, 1993.

Grant, P. N. Competition, collaboration and change: the emergence of California's new integrated delivery systems. *California Hospitals* Mar.–Apr. 1993, pp. 12, 31.

Healthcare Information and Management Systems Society (HIMSS) conference preview. *Hospitals and Health Networks,* 68(3):40–42, Feb. 5, 1994.

Helms, W. D. Testimony before the subcommittee on health committee on ways and means. State capacity to achieve health care reform. United States House of Representatives, Washington, DC, June 8, 1993.

Joint Commission for Accreditation of Healthcare Organizations. *Joint Commission Perspectives* 13(6):8, Nov.–Dec. 1993.

Joint Commission for Accreditation of Healthcare Organizations. *Joint Commission Perspectives.* Special issue on the 1994 accreditation manual for hospitals, 1994, p. 15.

Jones, W. J., and Mayerhofer, J. J. Regional health care systems: implications for health care reform. *Managed Care Quarterly* 2(1):31–44, 1994.

Lewin-VHI, Inc. Managed care: does it work? A report prepared for R. Atlas, D. Kennell, D. Sockel, and L. Lewin. Chicago, American Hospital Association, Jan. 27, 1993.

Managed Care Week, Integrated Trends for Managed Care Plans 4(16):2, May 2, 1994.

Minnesota's Integrated Service Networks. *Integrated Healthcare Report* July 1993, p.14.

Morrison, J. I. Railways of the nineties. *Healthcare Forum Journal* Mar.–Apr. 1994, pp. 30–34.

National Committee on Quality Assurance. *Health Plan Employer Data Information Set and Users' Manual,* Version 2.0, Washington, DC: NCQA, 1993.

Shortell, S. M. Creating organized delivery systems: the barriers and facilitators. *Journal of the Foundation of the American College of Healthcare Executives* 38(4):447–66, Winter 1993.

Welch, H. G., Miller, M. E., and Welch, W. P. Physician profiling: an analysis of inpatient practice patterns in Florida and Oregon. *New England Journal of Medicine* 330(9):607–12, Mar. 3, 1994.

Chapter Three

How to Set Up, Structure, Operate, and Develop Case Management

Chapter 3 sets forth the groundwork needed to set up a case management program, regardless of setting or of specific organizational strengths, weaknesses, and corporate culture. The chapter is divided into 10 main sections that delineate both case management theory and specific institutional examples.

The first few sections cover ways to introduce the case management concept, foster multidisciplinary program development, and clarify the definition of case management. Subsequent sections discuss suggested procedures for setting up a case management department, the importance of ensuring evolutionary program development, approaches to determining organizational structure and staffing needs, and the potential for applying case management beyond the acute care setting. The chapter concludes with advice on asking the right questions, measuring the impact of case management, and enhancing internal and external communication and marketing efforts.

Introducing the Case Management Concept

Change is an unpopular phenomenon, and in most instances introduction of the case management concept requires revising old ways of organizing, coordinating, providing, and measuring care. Although most administrative, clinical, and medical staff know in general that change is on the way, they can benefit from hearing the message again, particularly when different disciplines hear it simultaneously.

One way to introduce the concept of case management and justification for it is to use an outside consultant who has knowledge about the approach and experience with organizations that have already undergone substantial change in health care financing and delivery. First-hand observation of the success of case management in other settings can be more credible than the same observation made from within the organization. Also, a consultant can talk with a large and diverse group of people within an organization. In contrast, a site visit to a facility where case management is in place is limited to those who make the trip.

Although a good consultant may successfully introduce the case management concept, he or she is no substitute for an internal champion, that is, the individual within the organization who acts as a catalyst for change. Generally, an insider is best positioned to offer ongoing assistance with implementation, coordination, and troubleshooting.

Multidisciplinary Program Development

Any new concept involving health care professionals in different disciplines has the greatest chance for success if the people who will be affected have a role both in defining the problem and developing the solution. Total quality management (TQM) principles are very relevant in this respect.

For example, one New England community hospital that wanted to introduce the case management concept involved senior administrators (the president, chief operating officer, chief financial officer, and vice-presidents for managed care and patient services); key physicians; and utilization review, discharge planning, social service, and quality assurance staff in discussions about the need to revamp existing strategy and operations. The hospital's senior management did not issue an edict for change but instead took time to focus on processes of care. A diverse group of 15 people learned collectively and in individual sessions with an outside consultant that they needed to come up with a better way to manage patient care, integrate hospital and physician responsibilities, and produce and use data relating to cost and quality of care. After a three-month period of discussion and problem definition, the multidisciplinary group consensus was to implement a case management program.

During the discussion period, the group focused on the changing health care environment before it examined internal systems. Another motivating technique was to generate and review data comparing the hospital with its competitors and physicians with their peers. Only after the group understood the *what* and *why* of case management did it address the *how*.

Clarity of Definition

The concept of case management is not easy to understand. As explained in chapter 1, historically the term has had a plethora of applications (nursing case management, geriatric case management, catastrophic case management, and case management for mental health and substance abuse patients, and so forth).

In fact, institutions such as the Robert F. Kennedy Medical Center in Hawthorne, California, and the Strong Memorial Hospital in Rochester, New York, are more comfortable with the terms *care management* and *collaborative care*, respectively (*Hospital Case Management* 1993e). Keep in mind, however, that collaborative care also has different meanings in different settings. At New

England Medical Center, it means multidisciplinary collaboration, but at Carondelet St. Mary's Hospital and Health Center, it means provider/client collaboration.

Not only is the variety of applications of the term *case management* confusing, the possibilities and limitations of the function are puzzling. For example, does case management follow the patient, even if he or she moves out of the location where care or education was originally provided and into the continuum of care rendered in other settings? Or is the scope of case management limited to the organization that initially provided the care? Two institutions have become pioneers in taking their case management programs beyond the walls: Carondelet St. Mary's Hospital and Health Network in Tucson, Arizona (the case study in in chapter 7), and Daniel Freeman Memorial Hospital in Inglewood, California (*Hospital Case Management* 1993a and 1993b).

To add to the confusion over definition, case management is one of several popular concepts often referred to interchangeably (Crummer and Carter 1993). For example, clinical paths, critical paths, CareMapping® (Zander 1992), and outcomes measurement are *tools* that can be used to accomplish case management. They are not synonymous with case management. Brief descriptions of some of these tools are provided in figure 3-1; also see figure 3-2 for a sample clinical path.

A third definitional problem with the term *case management* is that it may replace, incorporate, and/or enhance utilization review, discharge planning, and social service. Quality assurance, although related to case management, is usually maintained as a separate activity.

Becoming familiar with different types of case management programs will help facilitate focus on the specific goals of a particular organization. Once the goals are clarified, choosing the right approach will be easier.

Steps to Introducing Case Management

The introduction of case management is a process, not an act. Steps in the process need a logical sequence, developed to increase the likelihood of ultimate success. Figure 3-3 (p. 34) lists the steps taken to introduce case management in a hospital that was not at the time using such tools as clinical paths and caremapping. Although the formal introduction of a physician component is shown as step 7, physician involvement in discussions began at the outset and continued throughout the process. (See the case study in chapter 5 for a more detailed description of how these steps were implemented.)

Many organizations have encountered a major stumbling block in determining the right sequence of steps. If they have already spent time and resources developing tools to facilitate, measure, and monitor the delivery of care, they may attempt to use the tools as the foundation for case management. Tools are tools, however, and they do not replace a comprehensive case management program complete with goals, structure, and staffing.

Figure 3-1. Tools and Techniques to Facilitate Case Management

Case management is a process, not to be confused with tools and techniques that can accomplish agreed-on goals.

Tool	Application
Algorithm	A decision tree for the clinical management of a specific diagnosis or patient undergoing a particular procedure
Benchmarking	A process for measuring an organization's product or pattern of service and comparing it to the "best practice" of high-quality institutions. The goal of benchmarking is to emulate the highest quality to improve.
CareMapping®	Introduced in 1991 by the Center for Case Management in Natick, MA, CareMaps® show multidisciplinary staff actions against a time line as well as key interventions necessary to produce stated outcomes (Zander, 1991 and 1992).
Clinical Indicators	Sometimes called flags, these are clinical occurrences that may indicate a problem with quality. Indicators may include a threshold beyond which there is an assumption of a quality problem. For example, a patient admitted for a normal delivery who began to show signs of infection would fall into this category.
Clinical Path	A provider-specific document that outlines key elements of the day-to-day care required by a typical patient with a particular diagnosis. Clinical paths may be developed to show current practice, or they may incorporate agreed-on "best practice" and target length of stay. Other terms used are *critical path, clinical pathway, care map, clinical map.* (See figure 3-2 for an example of a clinical path.)
Guideline	The recommended method for managing a particular condition. Guidelines are generally boundaries, not strict standards, that are meant to guide but not require a particular course of action.
Outcomes Measurement	An outcome is the result of a particular intervention, sometimes measured in terms of length or quality of life. Outcomes research or outcomes measurement seeks to compare the results of different treatment options.
Practice Parameters	Tools for clinical decision making based on scientific research, expert opinion, and other sources. Other terms are clinical practice guidelines or practice policies. Practice parameters are clinically focused and disease- or procedure-oriented.
Protocol	A document specifying the care that is to be provided to a patient undergoing a particular treatment. Protocols are often used in clinical research. They are strict management directives and more binding than guidelines.
Standard	A criterion of required practice that actual care is expected to meet. A standard implies unanimity of opinion regarding management of a condition.
Standard Treatment Protocol	An organization-specific document on which there is consensus, and that expands on a clinical path, providing detailed information on each aspect of the management of a patient with a particular diagnosis.

Sources: American Hospital Association. *Hospital Technology Special Report* 12(7):appendix c, June 1993; Zander, K. What's new in managed care and case management. *The New Definition* 6(2):1–2, Spring–Summer 1991; and Zander, K. Quantifying, managing, and improving quality: I, how CareMaps® link CQI to the patient. *The New Definition* 7(2):1–3, 1992.

Figure 3-2. Sample Clinical Path (Adult Appendectomy without Evidence of Peritonitis)

	Emergency/preop	First 24 hours postop	48 hours postop/discharge
Consults	Anesthesia		
Tests	Complete blood count with differential Electrolytes Urinalysis		Complete blood count
Treatments	IV fluids Weight	Heparin lock IV Check incision Abdominal dressing change as needed Cough & deep breathe with vital signs	D/C heparin lock Check incision Abdominal dressing change as needed Cough & deep breathe with vital signs
Assessment	Vital signs q 1–2 hours Weight	Vital signs q 2 hours Assess patient's pain q 2 hours, consider patient-reported pain assessment findings	Vital signs q 4–8 hours Assess patient's pain q 4–8 hours, consider patient-reported pain assessment findings
Medications	IV antibiotics, first dose within 2 hours preop After diagnosis established, IV Demerol 100 mg q 3 hours or IV Morphine 10 mg q 3–4 hours	Continue IV antibiotics Continue IV analgesics for 12 hours postop; switch to oral analgesic of choice when patient able to tolerate oral intake Adjust dose of analgesic if pain level is reported by patient as being "3" or higher	D/C antibiotics Continue oral analgesic Adjust dose of analgesic if pain level is reported by patient as being "3" or higher
Activity	Assist with care Out of bed with help	Ambulate with assistance Out of bed with help	Self-care Ambulate independently
Nutrition	Nothing by mouth	Clear liquid to full liquid	Regular diet
Elimination		Check bowel sounds	Check for bowel movement; may take milk of magnesia as needed at home
Teaching	General pre- and postop teaching Provide patient with education and information about pain control Develop with patient plan for pain control	Instruct patient in use of numeric pain self-assessment tool	Review discharge instructions Provide written discharge instructions that include details of pain management, including: • Specific drugs to be taken • Frequency of drug administration • Potential side effects of the medication • Potential drug interactions • Specific precautions to follow when taking the medication (e.g., physical activity limitations, dietary restrictions) • Name of individual to notify about pain problems and other postoperative concerns
Psychosocial	Patient/family support	Patient/family support	Patient/family support
Discharge planning	Admission assessment Continuing care as needed		Home health referral as needed

Source: Reprinted, with permission, from P. Spath. *Clinical Paths: Tools for Outcomes Management.* Chicago: American Hospital Publishing, 1994, p. 13.

Figure 3-3. Suggested Sequence of Steps for Developing Case Management

1. Acknowledge problems
2. Understand concept
3. Agree on goals
4. Decide on structure
5. Hire/designate department director
6. Cross-train staff
7. Integrate physician component
8. Develop tools to measure impact
9. Develop and use tools to facilitate case management
10. Expand program

Note: See chapter 5 for more details on how the steps were carried out.
Source: Reprinted, with permission, from The Malden Hospital, Malden, MA, 1994.

Evolutionary Program Development

In planning for implementation and development of case management, health professionals can benefit from the experiences of others. There is no "quick fix." The most reputable case management programs in the country contend that they will never be finished, that they will continue to evolve and change. There are good examples of evolving programs both within integrated systems (Sharp HealthCare, the subject of the chapter 8 case study), in tertiary facilities (Stanford University Hospital), and in organizations that anticipate becoming part of larger health care networks.

The Malden Hospital in Malden, Massachusetts (chapter 5), introduced case management at a time when the acute hospital and other subsidiaries of the holding company (that is, nursing home, home care) were still independent and not yet formally linked to other providers of care. The hospital and physicians knew they were in a transition mode. Although they did not know into which regional system they would ultimately fit, they saw no need to wait to improve the management of patient care in the existing delivery system.

At the outset, Malden combined the separate departments of utilization review, social service, and discharge planning into a single new case management department. A new director of case management was recruited from outside the organization. The utilization review and discharge planning staff, all of whom had nursing backgrounds, were cross-trained and assigned to each of the active physicians. Social service staff within the case management department provided consultation services as needed.

The concentration during year 1 was on acute inpatient care. The case managers worked closely with physicians to better manage the processes for admission, concurrent management of care, discharge, and postdischarge activities.

Within the acute hospital setting, case management achieved measurable success. "Administratively necessary days" decreased to 0, and the average Medicare charges declined by $5,000 per case. The case management staff achieved a very positive relationship with physicians and other professional staff, and patient satisfaction surveys provided favorable feedback.

In year 2 of case management at Malden, the program evolved beyond the acute inpatient setting. Impressed by the case managers' ability to solve problems, many hospital departments/programs asked for case management assistance in expediting patient care.

For example, the emergency department staff asked case managers to assist patients whose conditions did not warrant emergency treatment but who needed guidance in accessing care in a more appropriate setting. The ambulatory clinics asked the case managers to help educate patients and their families about support groups and to provide other assistance that clinic staff could not. The case managers were instrumental in setting up both an observation bed program and a new transitional care unit for patients no longer needing acute care. Most important, the hospital and selected physicians entered into several risk arrangements, including capitation, with two large managed health care plans. The success of case management gave them the confidence to manage their patients under risk-based reimbursement.

Although the case management program at Malden began in the acute inpatient setting, there was no intention of limiting the case managers' role. The hospital's holding company was also the parent corporation for a nursing home, and the expectation was that the case management program would formally extend into this institution as well. As the holding company began to acquire physician practices, the case management function was also expected to move into the physician office setting (Hospital Case Management 1994).

Organizational Structure and Staffing Needs

A number of factors must be taken into consideration when organizing a structure and staffing for case management. These range from matching institutional goals with the appropriate model of case management, to the type of care setting (tertiary care facilities or community care hospitals, for example), to whether integrated financing and delivery systems can facilitate case management.

There is no model structure or staffing pattern for case management that will work for all health care organizations. What works best is a program that has clear goals, is a high and visible organizational priority, has the commitment of the health professionals assuming the responsibility, and involves the entire organization. Some examples are described in the following subsections. Figures 3-4, 3-5, and 3-6 show sample organizational charts.

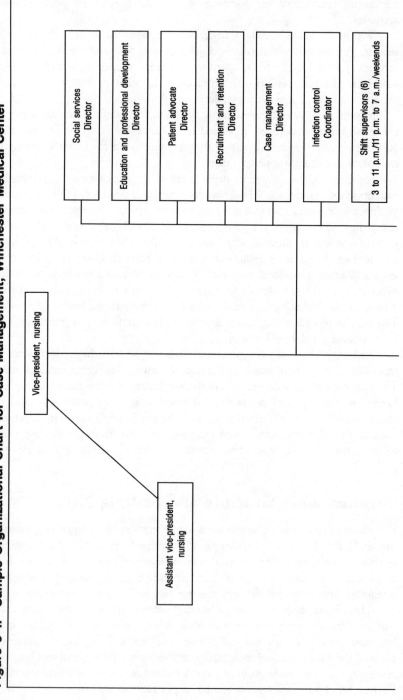

Figure 3-4. Sample Organizational Chart for Case Management, Winchester Medical Center

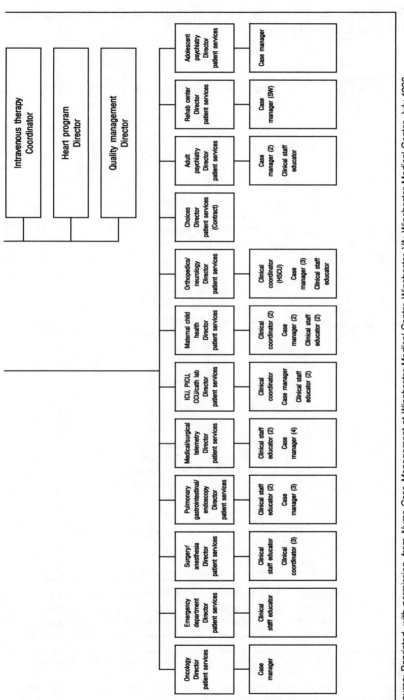

Source: Reprinted, with permission, from *Nurse Case Management at Winchester Medical Center.* Winchester, VA: Winchester Medical Center, July 1993.

Figure 3-5. Sample Organizational Chart for Case Management, Stanford University Hospital

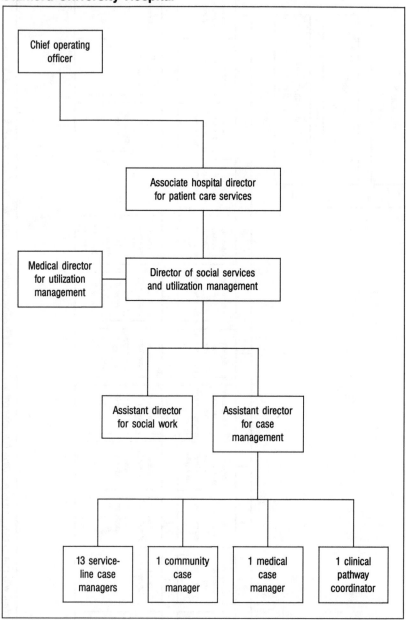

Note: Stanford University's case management was reorganized in September 1994 to report to a new quality support department.

Source: Reprinted, with permission, Stanford University Hospital, Department of Utilization Review and Social Work, Stanford, CA, Sept. 1994.

Figure 3-6. Sample Organizational Chart for Case Management, Baptist Memorial Hospital

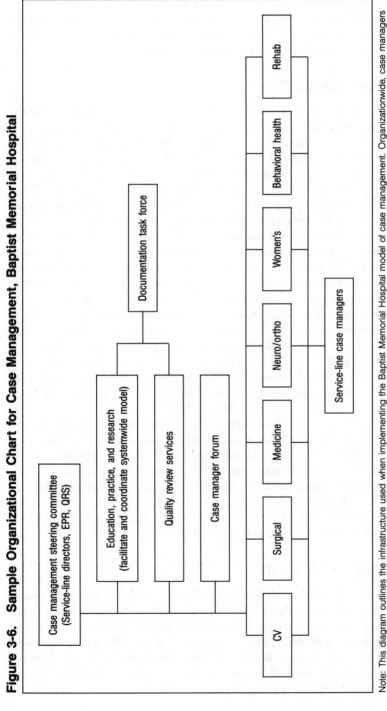

Note: This diagram outlines the infrastructure used when implementing the Baptist Memorial Hospital model of case management. Organizationwide, case managers report to their service-line director or administrator.

Source: Reprinted, with permission, from *Interdisciplinary Case Management*. 2nd ed. Memphis, TN: Baptist Memorial Hospital, August 1993.

Once the organization is clear about alternatives for case management, it can select the right fit between the various models and its own needs. A later section of this chapter poses a series of questions that can be helpful in making decisions related to structure and staffing.

Tertiary Care Facilities

Patients who require tertiary care have complex problems, and their care management requires efforts that differ from those needed in other settings.

New England Medical Center (NEMC) in Boston, Massachusetts, and The Center for Nursing Case Management in Natick, Massachusetts, were pioneers in the development of nursing case management in the 1980s (Grossman and Etheredge interviews 1994). The approach to case management at NEMC has been the model for many other providers. Etheredge distinguishes between cluster and serial configurations in the tertiary setting (Etheredge 1989).

In the *cluster* model, a patient is admitted by and discharged back to a physician or agency (for example, a nursing home)–care is provided in one unit of the hospital. In the *serial* model, patients receive care in more than one unit. Trauma patients, for example, may be transported by helicopter, admitted through the emergency department, and cared for in multiple units.

Although NEMC's case-based matrix and group practice concepts of collaborative care were used in both cluster and serial situations, there was variation in the application of the nursing case management concept. (The model has since evolved beyond what is described in Etheredge's book *Collaborative Care: Nursing Case Management*. For a description of the current model, see Zander's new book, *Managing Outcomes through Collaborative Care: The Application of Care Mapping and Case Management*.)

Another example of case management in a tertiary setting is the Baptist Memorial Hospital and Medical Center system in Memphis, Tennessee. Baptist has 1,900-plus beds on two campuses and 15 affiliated smaller hospitals. It uses an *interdisciplinary* model, rather than a program limited to one discipline; and its case managers, unlike the original nurse case managers at NEMC, *do not provide direct patient care*. The program is organized around a *product-line* or *service-line* structure. The cardiovascular service line in particular has been extremely successful (Duncan and Patterson 1993).

Community Hospitals

The Malden Hospital in Malden, Massachusetts, combined utilization review, discharge planning, and social service into a single department. The director of case management, recruited from an insurance company, reports directly to the executive vice-president, giving the program high visibility within the organization. Each case manager is assigned to an individual physician or physician group. Because the hospital is small, the case managers manage all of a physician's patients, regardless of diagnosis.

Integrated Financing and Delivery Systems

Some of the integrated financing and delivery systems have begun to deal with case management or care management across the continuum of care. Douglas Conrad, a professor in the Department of Health Services at the University of Washington in Seattle and an astute observer of these systems, distinguishes the importance of administrative and organizational–managerial integration from the "crucial" importance of the clinical integration of patient care. According to Conrad, "true vertically integrated care demands a system capacity to plan, deliver, monitor, and adjust the care of an individual over time." Furthermore, a system must be able to accomplish this same task for an entire population over time (Conrad 1993).

Two California systems, Friendly Hills HealthCare Network in La Habra and Sharp HealthCare in San Diego, are well along in the development of their case management networks/programs. Their accomplishments are described briefly here, and additional information is provided in the respective case studies that constitute chapters 6 and 8.

Friendly Hills HealthCare Network is an integrated provider system based around a large, multispecialty group practice. The system is responsible for 100,000 prepaid patients, including 15,000 seniors. It is at full risk for system enrollees. Ninety-five percent of its revenue is derived from 26 fully capitated managed care contracts. There are 150 providers at eleven office sites and one 297-bed hospital.

The case management network at Friendly Hills was developed at the corporate level by the vice-president, education, and is headed by a clinical nurse specialist (CNS). Both CNSs and geriatric nurse practitioners perform case management. The program goal is to apply a case management process in order to optimize the patient's functional and self-care abilities, prevent complications, facilitate system access to services and communication with the health care team, and coordinate appropriate utilization of resources (Brown 1994).

Sharp is a regional system of 5 hospitals, 14 clinics, 7 group practices, 5 skilled nursing facilities, an insurance product, and special services (Flower 1993). Case management existed before the components of Sharp became a system, and the current challenge is to modify the program to meet enrollee needs.

Sharp is either using or exploring three case management roles. For enrollees who need basic health management, prevention and wellness staff assist primary care providers. For enrollees with an acute or chronic diagnosis, a case manager may be assigned to ensure that access to care is timely, and that care is delivered according to clinical maps for treatment and resource use. The scope of responsibility includes the acute episode as well as the events prior to and following that event.

A small percentage of hospitalized enrollees—the more complex cases—cannot be managed by a clinical guideline or map. For these patients, service-line–specific case managers coordinate care, working closely with primary care providers and other care givers who may previously have been involved with the enrollee.

Staffing Considerations

A number of factors should be considered in determining case management staffing patterns. Most depend on specific organizational needs and the type of case management program to be undertaken. Three issues—promoting from within versus recruiting from outside the organization, staff qualifications, and staff size—are touched on here.

Existing Staff versus Outside Recruits

The director of case management sets the expectation and tone in terms of staffing alternatives. Some institutions have promoted from within, asking a professional already known to the organization to learn new techniques and assume new responsibilities. Others have recruited from the outside.

Again there is no one right way. Historically, some hospitals have felt that promotion from within has a disadvantage not easy to overcome. For example, because case management is a relatively new concept, the staff currently working in utilization review, discharge planning, social service, quality assurance, and nursing positions—likely candidates for the case management department head position—may not know how to do it. They also may have difficulty learning the job and teaching others.

Until fairly recently, the opportunities for learning case management have been limited and specific to individual professions, making continuing education difficult. For both reasons, lack of skill and lack of opportunities to learn, many organizations have looked outside for a case management director, turning to managed care plans, insurance companies, and utilization review firms. For case management staff below the director level, however, a solid argument can be made for retraining existing staff. (Appendix A at the back of this book contains a suggested curriculum for case manager education.)

Success will depend both on individuals' abilities to learn new techniques and on their working relationships with physicians and multiple departments. Staff who already have good relationships can quickly build on them.

Qualifications

Staff qualifications vary, depending on the program. A majority of organizations with case management designate professionals with a nursing background to perform the case management role. Tertiary facilities and some systems use registered nurses (RNs) trained as clinical nurse specialists. Some organizations require case management certification (Certification of Insurance Rehabilitation Specialist Commission 1992). Nurse practitioners may also be used for specific populations, such as geriatric clients. Community hospitals and ambulatory-based programs have successfully trained licensed practical nurses (LPNs).

Equally as important as clinical background and educational level is familiarity with alternative settings and community resources. Personal ability to interact with many people and to successfully solve complicated problems also is essential. (Figure 3-7, the case manager's creed, is a humorous look at the qualifications needed; figures 3-8, 3-9, 3-10, and 3-11 (pp. 44–54) contain sample job descriptions.)

Size

The size of the case management staff generally follows one of three patterns. Some organizations use a direct case manager/patient or case manager/enrollee ratio. Others assign case managers to physicians and take into consideration both the number of physicians per case manager and the number of patients or enrollees per physician. Finally, where product-line or service-line case management is focused on an inpatient unit, there may be a target ratio of case managers/unit, taking into account both beds per unit and average daily occupancy.

Figure 3-7. The Case Manager's Creed

To be a case manager, one must be courteous, diplomatic, caring, shrewd, persuasive, assertive, creative, supportive, understanding, responsible, slow to anger, adaptable, a Sherlock Holmes, a motivator, up-to-date, good-looking, have a good memory, acute business judgment, emotional stability, and be the embodiment of virtue, but with a good working knowledge of sin and evil in all its forms. ∗∗∗ A case manager must understand insurance, electricity, chemistry, physiology, mechanics, architecture, physics, bookkeeping, banking, merchandising, selling, shipping, contracting, claims adjusting, law, medicine, real estate, horse trading, and human nature. ∗∗∗ A case manager must be a coordinator, clinician, coach, therapist, educator, consumer advocate, and administrator. ∗∗∗ A case manager must be a mind reader, a hypnotist, and an athlete, must be acquainted with machinery of all types and materials of all kinds, and must know the current price of everything from a shoestring to a skyscraper, an aspirin to an amputation. They must know all, see all, and tell nothing, and be everywhere at the same time. ∗∗∗ They must satisfy the claims manager, the claims examiners, the home office claims department, the underwriting department, the supervisors, the solicitor, the insured, the claimant and the state industrial commission.

Source: ©1992 Nursefinders, Chicago, IL. Reprinted, with permission.

Figure 3-8.   Case Manager Job Description, The Malden Hospital

I. Job Description—Case Manager

Responsible to:

The case manager works under the direction and supervision of the chairperson of the clinical case management committee or his/her designee(s) and the director of case management.

Qualifications:

The case manager must:

1. Possess the knowledge in medical and allied health sciences necessary to apply criteria to the medical record with respect to patient needs for medical and health care.

2. Be knowledgeable about medical terminology, levels of care, treatment modalities, and the present health care delivery system, both hospital and community based.

3. Demonstrate the ability to make highly competent professional judgments and decisions.

4. Possess a high degree of skill in human relations with the ability to deal effectively on a one-to-one and group basis with physicians, nursing staff, administration, and other hospital department staff with whom he or she interacts.

5. Understand the formal and informal organizational structure and have the ability to relate effectively.

6. Demonstrate a desire and willingness to maintain and upgrade professional skills and education by attending and participating in relevant meetings, programs, and seminars.

Responsibilities and Duties:

1. Promote an understanding of case management:

   a. Maintaining familiarity with laws, regulations, and interpretation of utilization review and discharge planning.

   b. Remaining up-to-date on changes in regulations, policies, and procedures.

   c. Disseminating related material in a meaningful way to the chairperson of the clinical case management committee and to other appropriate hospital staff, including physicians.

   d. Monitoring utilization of clinical practice for determining covered case and length-of-stay parameters.

Figure 3-8. (Continued)

2. Conduct the case management program by:

    a. Following the policies and procedures as outlined in the case management manual.

    b. Referring all questionable utilization cases to a physician adviser for discussion and decision.

    c. Reviewing inpatient case every 24 hours. Providing utilization review in the inpatient, emergency department, and clinic settings as needed.

    d. Monitoring the patient's medical record to ascertain change of diagnosis or condition, arrival at apparent plateau, and present and future treatment plan.

    e. Maintaining daily relationship with physician case load.

    f. Collecting, recording, and maintaining all information gathered during the case management process.

    g. Following the established procedures in regard to denial of benefits notice.

    h. Maintaining reports of reviews conducted and length-of-stay denials.

3. Perform discharge assessment and planning functions by:

    a. Initiating the discharge planning assessment at the time of admission.

    b. Maintaining a comprehensive collaborative relationship with the patient, family, physician, payer, and health care team as to disposition needs and issues.

    c. Referring to social services any cases requiring consultation due to substance abuse, family dynamics, need for financial assistance, housing, maternal and child health concerns, cancer support, long-term placement, or health care proxy issues.

    d. Promoting a timely, cost-effective, efficient, and safe discharge plan to community services, including extended care, long-term care, or home health services.

    e. Providing appropriate clinical documentation concerning discharge information to the provider of postacute care.

    f. Maintaining federal and state regulations for the documentation of the discharge planning process.

    g. Monitoring discharge planning efficiency by a telephone follow-up within 48 hours of discharge.

    h. Collaborating with: the admitting office, medical records, patient accounts, administration, and patient care departments as needed to ensure effective and efficient communication of efforts and activities.

Professional levels:

Case manager 1: RN licensure
Case manager 2: LPN licensure

Source: Reprinted, with permission, from The Malden Hospital, Malden, MA, 1994.

**Figure 3-9. Specialty Case Manager Job Description and
Performance Standards, Sharp Memorial and Cabrillo Hospitals**

Title: Specialty case manager

Reports to: Program manager, clinical manager, and regional director

Position purpose: This position is responsible for the coordination of all systems/services
                   required for an organized, multidisciplinary team approach and assures
                   quality, cost-efficient care for the identified patient population.

Responsibilities:

1. Assessment, data collection, and analysis
   a. Obtains, reviews, and analyzes information in collaboration with the patient, family,
      significant other, health care team members, employers, legal representative, and
      claims/insurance personnel as indicated.
   b. Assesses the patient's clinical and psychosocial status, diagnosis, and current
      treatment plan.
   c. Assesses the patient/family/significant other needs related to the medical diagnosis,
      treatment providers, treatment options, financial resources, psychosocial needs, and
      discharge planning.

2. Establishment of goals and plans of care
   a. In collaboration with health care team members, sets patient-centered goals for
      individual patients/families/significant others.
   b. Utilizes tools and resources (that is, clinical pathways and data bases) to develop a
      comprehensive multidisciplinary plan of care.

3. Implementation
   a. Intervenes when variances occur in a patient's individualized treatment plan.
   b. Coordinates and evaluates the patients' and family's use of resources and services
      in a quality-conscious, cost-effective manner.
   c. Facilitates and collaborates with the health care team for timely discharge planning.
   d. Coordinates access to appropriate government and community programs and resources.

4. Evaluations and patient outcomes
   a. Monitors and evaluates short-term and long-term patient responses to therapeutic
      interventions, maintaining interdependent follow-up as necessary.
   b. Analyzes patterns of variance from the standardized clinical pathways and
      implements strategies to resolve them.
   c. Facilitates and/or participates in conferences that provide ongoing evaluation of
      interdisciplinary dynamics, goal attainment, and treatment plan revision.

5. Quality assurance/improvement
   a. Participates in quality assessment (QA)/quality improvement (QI) activities by
      evaluating patient care systems that may include standards, protocols, and
      documentation for efficiency, safety, and quality.
   b. Incorporates evaluative data in the provision of ongoing case management services.

6. Educator
   a. Ensures instruction to the patient and family based on identified learning needs.
   b. Assesses the family's knowledge base, health status expectations, and the potential
      for/or actuality of a family member acting as the primary care giver if necessary.
   c. Assists with the development of activities and methods to ensure information is
      articulated and disseminated to staff.

7. Communication, leadership, collaboration, consultant liaison
   a. Collaborates with the health care team, payers, community agencies, providers, and legal
      representatives to ensure continuity of the patient's care through all health care settings.

Figure 3-9. (Continued)

   b. Promotes effective communication among health care team members, including the patient, family, significant other, and payers.

   c. Participates in team meetings when indicated.

   d. Incorporates recommendations and/or services of interdisciplinary team members in plan of care.

   e. Uses interpersonal communication strategies with individuals, as well as groups of patients/families/significant others and staff that result in:

      —Achievement of intended outcomes

      —Others' expressed perception of acceptance/satisfaction

   f. Perceived by other health care workers as approachable when assisting in the achievement of established goals and objectives for improving clinical outcomes.

   g. Develops collaborative relationship with other departments/entities/external health care agencies to facilitate and support quality care.

   h. Acts as a resource on complex patient care activities.

   i. Establishes and maintains communication systems with individuals/agencies providing interdisciplinary care in the area of clinical expertise.

   j. Identifies and directly addresses issues that affect patient care outcomes; collaborates with appropriate providers to prevent recurrence of issues.

   k. Participates in service-line committees, cost quality committee, marketing/sales endeavors, and contracting.

8. Documentation

   a. Provides routine verbal and written documentation of the initial assessment and progress of the individual to the payer and/or appropriate others on a timely, regular basis.

   b. If appropriate, documents patient's progress on clinical pathways.

9. Community integration (discharge)

   a. Assists patient, family, and significant other on anticipating the needs and making plans for returning home or an alternative living site.

10. Professional responsibilities

   a. Plans for personal growth as related to professional goals based on self-assessment, evaluation, and feedback.

   b. Assumes responsibility for acquiring knowledge and experience to meet goals.

   c. Actively participates in professional organizations.

11. Financial issues

   a. Provides education, guidance, and recommendations to the payer regarding alternatives for care and services when appropriate.

   b. Utilizes strategies to manage the length of stay and resource utilization within the case-managed patient populations and document the results.

   c. Acts as a liaison between third-party payer, health care team, and patient, family, significant other.

   d. Coordinates with third-party payers the progress toward treatment goals and established criteria in the most cost-effective way.

Qualifications:

1. R.N., B.S.N. required.
2. M.S.N. preferred.
3. Three (3) years' clinical experience in related field.
4. One (1) year's experience in case management and/or similar role.
5. Current case management certification preferred.

(Continued on next page)

Figure 3-9.   (Continued)

Sharp Memorial and Cabrillo Hospitals Performance Standards

Position title: Specialty Case Manager

Date: November 22, 1993

Position purpose:

> This position is responsible for the coordination of all systems/services required for an organized, multidisciplinary team approach and assures quality, cost-efficient care for the identified patient population.

> The case manager functions as a contact person for patient, family, health care team members, employees, and claims/insurance personnel as necessary.

Performance standards:

1. Quality of care, 40%

   a. Assures that all designated patients within service line have individualized plan of care.

   b. Assures development of clinical pathway/algorithm protocols.

   c. Evaluates the quality and appropriateness of care by variance tracking and analysis.

   d. Implements a formal feedback survey to evaluate customer satisfaction (patients need to be surveyed).

2. Resource utilization/finance, 30%

   a. Assures appropriate use of patient care resources and monitors their financial impact to the service line.

   b. Actively negotiates payment plan for patient.

3. Leadership/communication/collaboration, 30%

   a. Provides leadership as evidenced by scores on Leadership Skill Inventory (score points).

   b. Demonstrates collaborative working relationships with all members of the health care team.

   c. Anticipates patient care issues and actively problem-solves utilizing CQI methodology and tools with health care team.

   d. Establishes ongoing communication and formal documentation systems to ensure that all members of health care team are informed.

Source: Reprinted, with permission, from Sharp HealthCare, San Diego, CA, copyright 1994.

Figure 3-10. Case Manager Job Description, Baptist Memorial Hospital

The Case Manager: Functions, Responsibilities, and Job Specifications

A new role and job position of case manager was developed in 1992. As a budget neutral process, the focus was on job and work redesign. Registered nurses from quality review services were merged and cross-trained with clinical nurse specialists and other qualified clinicians.

The functions and responsibilities of the case manager include the following key areas:

- Clinical management of patients to include coordination and brokering of services among the group practice members and coordination of services beyond the "hospital walls" as needed.

- Concurrent quality assessment and variance analysis

- Assisting patients in benefits management to include negotiation with third-party payers and agencies for recertification of alternative cost-effective levels of care

There are currently 27 case managers at Baptist Memorial Hospital—Medical Center and 17 at Baptist Memorial Hospital—East. They are assigned to specific, top-volume admitting physicians within the service lines in order to establish and maintain collaborative relationships.

Patients are divided among case managers based on the service line in which they are admitted, the physicians to whom they are assigned, and the working DRG, or care path, assigned to the patients.

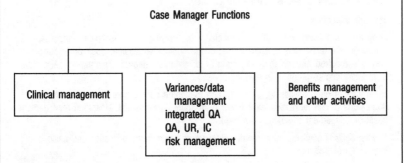

Case managers coordinate the care and service of selected patient populations across the continuum of illness; promote effective utilization; monitor health care resources; and assume a leadership role with the interdisciplinary team to achieve optimal clinical and resource outcomes.

Job Responsibilities

- Assesses, develops, implements, and monitors a comprehensive plan of care through an interdisciplinary team process in conjunction with the patient and family in internal and external settings.
  - Comprehensively assesses patients' goals as well as their biophysical, psychosocial, environmental, and discharge planning needs and financial status
  - Procures services and advocates on behalf of the patients and families for scarce resources
  - Acts as a liaison to posthospital care providers and community health resources

(Continued on next page)

Figure 3-10.   (Continued)

* On a concurrent basis assesses: appropriateness of the level of care; diagnostic testing and clinical procedures performed; quality and clinical risk issues; and documentation of medical record completeness. Reports all variances through the established case management and quality improvement processes.

  —As appropriate, reviews all patient admission data within the designated time frames to determine the suitability of the level of care in accordance with hospital-sanctioned ISDA criteria and/or other established criteria
  —Conducts quality monitoring activities according to established plans
  —Develops/revises tools for use in quality monitoring
  —Prepares specific data for reappointment and/or reappraisal

* Communicates continually with patients, families, medical staff, care givers, and third-party payers as necessary.

  —Relates utilization assessments needed to justify continued hospitalization and to obtain procedure precertification
  —Communicates with patients to ensure understanding of third-party payer guidelines and to arrange discharge planning referrals as ordered by patient's physicians

* Formulates, implements, and evaluates educational strategies for patients and families.

  —Facilitates or provides necessary patient and family education prior to admission, during hospital stay, and posthospital discharge as indicated

* Analyzes case management outcome data to identify and make recommendations within a designated service line.

* Develops and maintains a positive work climate and the overall team effort of the hospital.

* Performs other duties as assigned or directed.

Job Specifications

Knowledge and Education: Skill and proficiency in applying highly technical principles, concepts, and techniques that are central to the nursing profession. Such proficiency is normally acquired through the completion of an associate degree, diploma, baccalaureate, or masters degree program in nursing.

Experience: Skill in assessing, planning, and managing patient care as acquired through three years of clinical nursing experience in an acute care hospital. Utilization management/ quality management experience preferred.

Special Skills: Knowledge of computer software and hardware application and basic knowledge of statistics.

Interpersonal Requirements: Advanced communications and interpersonal skills with all levels of internal and external customers. This includes, but is not limited to: medical staff, patients and families, clinical personnel, support and technical staff, outside agencies, and members of the community. Interpersonal skills to obtain and interpret information appropriate to patient's needs and age as required for assessment, range of treatment, and patient care.

Orientation to the Case Manager Role

• ISDA criteria	4 hours	• Role of physician adviser	2 hours
• Levels of care	2 hours	• Variances and data	
• Medicare and third-party		management	2 hours
reimbursement	2 hours	• Negotiations skills	3 hours
• DRG optimization	16 hours	• Time management	4 hours

Source: Reprinted, with permission, from *Interdisciplinary Case Management.* 2nd ed. Memphis, TN: Baptist Memorial Hospital, August 1993.

Figure 3-11. Case Manager Job Description, Winchester Medical Center

Job Description	

Job Title: RN Case Manager   **Department:** Nursing
Reports to: Director of Patient Services

This job description is based on an evaluation of the position at the time this description was written. This job description will change from time to time as tasks, organization, and technology change. Accordingly, the employer reserves the unlimited right to revise all or any part of this job description and the essential functions of the job and to add or eliminate essential functions of any position. Designation of any job duty as an "essential function" is not intended as an assurance or guarantee that an employee has any right to perform the particular job duty, except as required by the employer.

Qualifications (physical requirements attached):

1. Current registered nurse licensure in the State of Virginia.
2. Bachelor of Science in Nursing preferred, or related collegiate courses.
3. Recent clinical experience of at least two years in the designated specialty area.
4. Demonstrated ability in the application of the nursing process to patient care in an acute care setting.

Temperament:

This position requires a person with a positive attitude who is pleasant and cooperative, displaying a professional demeanor with patients, families, physicians, and fellow employees. This position requires the ability to remain productive under stress.

		Performance Rating			
Percentage	Responsibility Area and Performance Standards	1 Does Not Meet Standards	2 Meets Standards	3 Generally Exceeds Standards	4 Outstanding
20%	C.A.R.E. • *Courtesy*—Consistently courteous to visitors, patients, and fellow employees whether speaking directly or by telephone. Routinely anticipates the needs of others and seeks opportunities to be courteous. • *Attitude*—Manner of dressing, body language, and verbal tone consistently communicates a positive professional and friendly image. Generally inspires confidence. Is always receptive to constructive feedback and coaching. • *Respect*—Consistently demonstrates respect for self, the work being done, and the needs and feelings of the patients and fellow workers. Always respects the rights and dignity of others. • *Enthusiasm*—Frequently seeks opportunities to make positive comments and encourage others. Encourages positive morale and enthusiasm among the WMC employee team.				

(Continued on next page)

Figure 3-11.   (Continued)

		Performance Rating			
Percentage	Responsibility Area and Performance Standards	1 Does Not Meet Standards	2 Meets Standards	3 Generally Exceeds Standards	4 Outstanding
45%	Clinical • Identifies appropriate patients/caseloads within designated specialty area requiring nurse case management interventions. • Assumes responsibility for ongoing assessment of patient care needs through frequent patient rounds and communication with clinical coordinators, clinical educators, direct nursing care givers, physicians, and other members of the health care team. • Assures the progress pathway/patient plan of care is initiated within 72 hours of admission, using appropriate patient goals/expected outcomes. • Collaborates with primary nurse in formulating plan of care using the nursing process in patient conferences and rounds. • Evaluates and collaborates with all members of the health care team to document patient status and variances, working toward achievement of patient goals/expected outcomes. • Establishes ongoing dialogue with the patient and/or family to determine if patient needs are being met. • Encourages nursing staff to participate in discharge planning rounds on a regular basis. • Effectively works with all members of the health care team to evaluate and update changes in the patient's plan of care. • Promotes safe, competent nursing care that follows the philosophy, policies and procedures, and nursing care standards of the Division of Nursing. • Collaborates with Social Work in identifying patient discharge needs, making appropriate referrals, and utilizing available community/regional resources. • Participates in the evaluation of patent care products. • Encourages nursing staff to utilize resources in a cost-effective manner.				

Figure 3-11. (Continued)

Percentage	Responsibility Area and Performance Standards	Performance Rating			
		1 Does Not Meet Standards	2 Meets Standards	3 Generally Exceeds Standards	4 Outstanding
25%	Leadership • Enhances understanding of the nurse case management process through availability and interactions with patients/family and all members of the health care team. • Serves as a liaison for the physician/nursing staff/ancillary departments to implement processing of the patient through the health care delivery system. • Engenders confidence of patients, staff, and community through appearance and behavior, and by serving as a positive role model. • Recognizes patient's rights by providing for confidentiality of patient information and demonstrates respect for patient's dignity. • Identifies professional goals and evaluates achievement. • Demonstrates an awareness of current trends that influence nursing practice. • Fulfills professional responsibilities by demonstrating accountability for nursing actions. • Exhibits openness to change and willingness to try new approaches as manifested in behavior. • Collaborates in establishing, maintaining unit goals, objectives, and evaluating progress toward their attainment. • Actively participates in unit, division, and hospital standing and ad hoc committees, as well as in special projects. • Promotes quality management by initiating/participating in unit-specific reviews and assists with quality monitoring. • Provides information to the director of patient services regarding nursing staff's clinical performance in the delivery of patient care. • Actively contributes to the review/revision/implementation of nursing standards of care, and policies and procedures for designated specialty area. • Performs other duties requested by manager.				

(Continued on next page)

Figure 3-11.   (Continued)

Percentage	Responsibility Area and Performance Standards	Performance Rating			
		1 Does Not Meet Standards	2 Meets Standards	3 Generally Exceeds Standards	4 Outstanding
10%	Education • Collaborates with nursing staff and other case managers to identify patient/family educational needs. • Encourages/educates nursing staff in use of various educational resources (for example, videos, flipcharts, pamphlets) to meet varied patient educational needs. • Collaborates with other case managers in the development of patient teaching plans and programs for their designated specialty area and for the Division of Nursing. • Reviews patient and/or family educational needs with the primary nurse and monitors documentation of teaching/learning on the Progress Pathway. • Is accountable for identifying own learning needs and seeking sources of information. • Actively participates in and attends educational opportunities, meetings, workshops, and seminars relative to need for additional information. • Identifies individual staff education needs and collaborates with the clinical educator for intervention. • Uses current knowledge and skills to promote safe patient care and to identify potentially unsafe practices.				

Source: Reprinted, with permission, from *Nurse Case Management at Winchester Medical Center*. Winchester, VA: Winchester Medical Center, 1994.

Case Management beyond the Acute Episode of Illness

Hospitals and systems that are setting up case management programs need to consider both their current situations and the possibility that they will become part of a fully integrated health care financing and delivery system. Potential applications for case management beyond the acute inpatient setting—in the emergency department, in ambulatory settings, in physicians' offices, and in home settings—are described in the following subsections.

Case Management in the Emergency Department

Ironically, emergency departments can be the point of both first and last resort. Individuals without health insurance coverage or those with coverage who do not follow health plan rules may use the emergency department instead of a primary care physician, as well as for true emergencies. As employee cost sharing increases, however, more and more people are using the emergency department when they should, that is, for life-threatening emergencies.

In any event, many who seek emergent care can be encouraged to properly access the health care system. Once the clinical professionals have completed their triage and assessment, case managers can divert patients to more appropriate settings and resources, often soothing angry tempers. Case managers also can teach emergency department staff to problem-solve and to refer patients to home care, social agencies, and other services when necessary.

Case Management in Ambulatory Settings

As inpatient care shifts to outpatient care, ambulatory staff will deal with cases that are more complex than they have treated previously. Clinical needs may be easier to meet than related social needs. Again, case managers can help direct patients to the appropriate points of service and also educate staff.

Case Management in Physician Offices

As with ambulatory settings, the diversion from inpatient to outpatient care will mean physician offices are asked to respond in different ways. Case managers can help office staff to courteously and appropriately direct patients and families.

Case Management in Home Settings

The decrease of both hospital utilization and length of stay means that more people will recuperate for longer periods of time at home. The need for that "know-it-all" who can ease the transition from institutional to home setting is key. In maternity care, for example, as the length of stay for normal vaginal deliveries shortens, mothers will go home sooner. Much of the education and support they previously had received in the hospital will be given at home.

Winchester Medical Center in Winchester, Virginia, has also had good results with a community-based nursing case management program that grew out of the original hospital-based program (Zerull 1994). The expanded program is targeted at patients with such chronic conditions as congestive heart failure, chronic obstructive pulmonary disease, angina, and diabetes. More recently, adult psychiatric and maternal and infant populations have been included.

Many of the patients who receive case management services at Winchester do not qualify for home health care, but in the opinion of the direct care givers, they are not self-sufficient enough to return home without assistance. The case management option for postdischarge follow-up helps increase patient and family confidence in managing complex needs and often prevents unnecessary readmission.

Asking the Right Questions

As health care providers assess their options for the structure and staffing of case management programs, they should look carefully at the experiences of those who have been there before them. (Appendix B contains suggestions for accessing information on other providers.) At the very least, the following questions should be addressed:

- *Does the organization provide or expect to provide the full continuum of care, including education and wellness, ambulatory care, acute inpatient care, skilled nursing care, home care, rehabilitation, and so on?*
- *If the organization is not currently part of a network, what are its plans and timing for becoming part of a more comprehensive system?*
- *Is there a corporate or staff resource who can serve as the internal case management visionary or champion?*
- *Does the top level of the organization have interest in, and commitment to, case management?*
- *Do physicians understand and support the case management concept?*
- *Will the case manager function as a facilitator of care that is provided by others, or will he or she provide direct care?*
- *Will the target group for case management be determined by formula, judgment, or a combination of the two?* Figure 3-12 contains the screens used by Winchester Medical Center to identify high-risk patients who might benefit from case management. The methods used by Friendly Hills HealthCare Network and Carondelet St. Mary's Hospital and Health Center are described in chapters 6 and 7 respectively.

Figure 3-12. Winchester Medical Center's Screens for Identifying High-Risk Patients Who Might Benefit from Case Management

---

Universal Indicators for High-Risk Proposed Screens

1. Any patient admitted from a nursing home, chronic care facility, foster home health agency, or is active with a community agency.

2. Any patient whose condition will affect his or her ability to return home, including those requiring "high tech" care.

3. Any patient with a history of frequent readmission or hospitalization within 15 days of last discharge.

4. Any patient exhibiting prolonged fear and/or anxiety about recommended medical procedures.

5. Any patient who is a suspected victim of abuse, neglect, or violence.

6. Any patient with identified problems whose medical compliance hinges on adequate housing and/or physical conditions.

7. Any patient whose conditions will necessitate a change in employment and/or family roles or quality of life.

8. Any patient whose condition has resulted in identified problems which will negatively affect self-image, appearance, physical, and/or sexual functioning.

9. Any patient whose identified personal, family, or financial problems directly affect care, treatment, and medical compliance.

10. Any patient or patient's family who exhibits behavior that is disruptive to treatment.

11. Any patient who resides outside the normal service area and has an illness that will affect his or her ability to return home.

12. Any patient admitted for treatment as a result of a catastrophic event.

13. Any patient in the terminal stages of illness or is a candidate for organ transplant.

14. Any patient who is known to, or suspected of, chemical abuse or addiction.

15. Those patients 75 years of age or older and/or living alone.

Source: Reprinted, with permission, from *Nurse Case Management at Winchester Medical Center.* Winchester, VA: Winchester Medical Center, 1994.

- *Will the case manager follow the patient and family beyond the walls of the organization in which the contact was made?* For example, if hospitalization in an acute facility precipitated the assignment of a case manager to a patient, can that case manager follow the patient into other settings such as home care, nursing home, rehabilitation facility, or ambulatory settings?

- *Is it important for a patient to keep the same case manager regardless of the cause for entry into the health care system, or will the patient be assigned to different case managers depending on the specific health care need?* For example, some hospitals have DRG-specific case managers, so patients with multiple problems may interact with several different case managers who coordinate their activities.

- *Can the organization cross-train existing staff for case management, or will it look for outside expertise?* In times when the health care delivery system is changing rapidly and staffing needs are shrinking, case management may offer opportunities for professional growth.
- *Who will pay for case management?* When the function is integrated into the inpatient function, the cost may be included in hospital departmental budgets. If the case management program is ambulatory or community-focused, it may make sense to seek payer reimbursement under capitation. As described in chapter 7, Carondelet St. Mary's took such an approach.

Measuring the Impact of Case Management

An important part of all case management programs should be incorporation of a methodology to evaluate its impact. Patricia Cloonan, Ph.D., R.N., a faculty member at Georgetown University School of Nursing in Washington, D.C., and Donna Havens, Ph.D., R.N., assistant professor of nursing at Duke University School of Nursing in Durham, North Carolina, offered many interesting ideas on evaluation at the First Southeastern Case Management Network Conference held in Durham in October 1993 (*Hospital Case Management* 1993f).

Impact evaluation can be divided into five areas: staff satisfaction, patient and family satisfaction, quality improvement, improvement of interdisciplinary communication/collaboration, and financial impact. These areas can be measured by surveys, TQM tools, and other methods incorporated into the program design. These areas are described in the following subsections.

Staff Satisfaction

Case management can be expected to improve the satisfaction of both the staff directly responsible for the job, as well as for those whose work may be made easier by the existence of a case management program. If the program is working smoothly, physicians and their office staffs should also have positive feedback.

Patient and Family Satisfaction

Although the case management concept may be new to patients and their families, if the program is effective they should experience efficient and well-coordinated delivery of care during the episode of illness and leave with a good understanding of what comes next. For example, Carondelet St. Mary's, a pioneer with case management beyond the walls, has reported the results of its research on the client impact of case management for high-risk adults. From a client perspective, as the nurse case manager grows as "insider expert," the case manager–client relationship goes through three phases: bonding, working, and changing (Lamb and Stempel 1994). Patient surveys are an effective tool for measuring response and eliciting suggestions to continually improve this relationship.

Improved Quality

Some of the ways in which case management can be expected to improve the quality of patient care include reduction in length of stay, readmission rate, and administratively necessary days; increased uniformity of treatment; increased frequency and effectiveness of patient education; and increased ability to measure and correct any aspects of care that vary from expectations. These indicators can be measured at different points in time. Although it is difficult to know if case management alone causes improved outcomes, the measurements provide a good picture of change.

Improved Interdisciplinary Communication and Collaboration

Although the communication and collaboration indicator is somewhat more difficult to measure than the others, organizations can assess the development of collaborative practice groups and the creation of multidisciplinary action plans. At The Malden Hospital in Malden Massachusetts, the development of a case management department stimulated both the nursing division and the emergency department staff respectively to change their structures and approaches to dealing with patients and physicians. (See the case study in chapter 5 for more detail.)

Financial Impact

Case management can have a financial impact by improving resource use; reducing staff absenteeism, turnover, and vacancies; decreasing wait time for tests and procedures; and decreasing denials by insurance companies. Both Stanford University Hospital and The Malden Hospital obtained major cost savings by implementing case management.

Internal and External Communication and Marketing

As is true of measurement of the impact of case management, communication and marketing for the program are ongoing processes. The organizations most successful with case management share information internally and externally throughout planning, development, and implementation.

Internal Communication

Internal communication about case management is important for a number of reasons. First, it ensures that everybody understands the concept. Case management is not a black-and-white process and is likely to cause confusion and concern for those who have never worked with such a system. By talking about it—what it is, what it is not, and how it fits into the ongoing operations of a specific organization—the mystery is dissolved early on.

Next, open discussion encourages input. Because case management can take whatever shape is appropriate for a particular organization/health care setting, open discussion encourages various medical and nonmedical staff to share ideas, many of which can be incorporated into the final concept.

Finally, those affected want part of the action. As case management becomes a reality, particularly as a helpful and nonthreatening activity, those on whom it has impact will want to participate. In The Malden Hospital example mentioned earlier and described at length in chapter 5, case management started with acute inpatient care and expanded to cover other departments. Potential users, as well as the case management department itself, shaped the program. As the case managers' reputations as problem solvers grew, their services and approach became contagious.

External Communication

Health care providers or systems with case management programs in place have an advantage over other providers if they can describe what they do, document their achievements, and communicate their accomplishments to those who use and purchase care (patients and their families, referring physicians and their office staffs, managed care plans, employers, and other health care providers). The following subsections suggest target audiences and different marketing techniques for internal and/or external activities.

Target Audience

For patients and their families, the experience of interfacing with the health care delivery system can be a bewildering, frightening, and disruptive experience. Particularly unsettling are unexpected emergencies, the potential for large bills, and now so-called alternatives to inpatient care that might convey the notion of less expensive but less effective settings.

As a single focal point for information about care at all levels—preventive, outpatient, inpatient, subacute, rehabilitation, long-term, and home-based care—the case manager can counteract that negative impression. Good communication can convey the more correct impression that care in multiple settings has been thoughtfully planned and linked together.

The case manager can also provide health education. As reimbursement moves toward payment by capitation, the goal of keeping people healthy and out of the delivery system becomes more important. An effective case manager with a strong bond with patient and family can build on that relationship and convey preventive as well as prescriptive information. Finally, the case manager offers the patient and family the objectivity of an outside arbiter when and if there is disagreement and/or tension among family members.

Physicians
Although good case management programs are multidisciplinary, the case manager–physician relationship is critical and can determine the success or failure of a program. If the case manager develops a good working relationship with physicians and becomes the single focal point for information on medical and nonmedical issues, the physician has gained a valuable resource.

The relationship between case manager and physician office staff is also important. An effective case manager can assist office staffs with scheduling and coordination of tests and procedures. More important, he or she can be a valuable resource for both medical and nonmedical alternatives.

Managed Care Plans
Case management offers a marketing advantage in dealing with health plans, for several reasons. Until such time as insurers and providers are truly combined into integrated systems, plans will continue to shift risk to providers. Providers who can best control that risk will have a competitive advantage. For example, one community hospital that was historically risk-averse and protective about contractual relationships with managed health care plans altered its strategy after setting up a case management program. The institution actually sought out opportunities for risk sharing and even capitation because it knew that it could manage the patient care.

Employers
Employer decision making about health insurance should take into account not only the cost of different options but the provider networks that each plan offers. All things being equal, a provider with a case management program offers purchasers a better chance to provide cost-effective care than a provider without the program. The Malden Hospital (chapter 5 case study) used its case management program to distinguish itself from other neighboring hospitals and actively attempted to influence employer choice of health insurance. Employers saw that hospital's case management program as an innovative way to coordinate care — and ultimately to control cost.

Marketing Techniques

Described here are some ideas for marketing case management to internal and/or external audiences. Appendix B contains specific references.

• Frequent and public description of case management activities, using patient-specific examples of success. Internal, department head meetings and informational sessions for office managers are good ways to share such information.
• Brief descriptions of successful and difficult-to-resolve cases for medical staff grand rounds and for medical staff publications.

- Public interest stories in local newspapers, featuring patients and families who were satisfied with the assistance of the case manager. For example, a regional newspaper featured an article and picture of an elderly patient whose case manager had helped her return to her home instead of to a nursing home. After reading the article, many patients and families contacted the hospital about the "extra" service they could get—at no additional charge.
- Bulletin board displays on case management for patients, families, and visitors to use as an educational tool.
- Case management diagrams posted in patient rooms that give patients and families an explanation of the expected timetable for care. For example, Kennestone Hospital in Marietta, Georgia, and Anne Arrundel Medical Center in Annapolis, Maryland, display user-friendly diagrams in patient rooms so that patients and families have clear expectations about the course of care (*Hospital Case Management* 1993a). St. Vincent's Hospital and Medical Center in Portland, Oregon, uses "patient-oriented itineraries" that are written in multiple languages (*Hospital Case Management* 1993d).

Case managers can be their own best advocates. The better they do their jobs, the more problems they resolve; the more visible they are, the more people will ask for their help.

References and Bibliography

Brown, N., vice-president, education; Jacoby, A., cardiopulmonary clinical nurse; and Mumaw L., geriatric nurse practitioner. Telephone interviews with Friendly Hills Health-Care Network, La Habra, CA, Mar., Apr., May 1994.

Certification of Insurance Rehabilitation Specialist Commission. *Certification for Case Management*. Rolling Meadows, IL: Certification of Insurance Rehabilitation Specialist Commission, Sept. 1992.

Conrad, D. A. Coordinating patient care services in regional health systems: the challenge of clinical integration. *Journal of the Foundation of the American College of Healthcare Executives* 38(4):492, Winter 1993.

Crummer, M. B., and Carter, V. Critical pathways—the pivotal tool. *Journal of Cardiovascular Nursing* 7(4):30–37, July 1993.

Duncan, K., and Patterson, J. Enhancing outcomes with case management. *The Journal of Cardiovascular Management* 4(3):33–39, May–June 1993.

Etheredge, M. L. S., editor. *Collaborative Care: Nursing Case Management*. Chicago: American Hospital Publishing, 1989, pp. 27–29.

Etheredge, M. L. S. Telephone interview with director of nursing education, New England Medical Center, Boston, MA, Mar. 18, 1994.

Flower, J. Getting paid to keep people healthy. *Healthcare Forum Journal* 37(2):51-53, Mar.-Apr. 1993.

Grossman, J. Interview with president of New England Medical Center, Boston, MA, Jan. 6, 1994.

Hospital Case Management. To post or not to post: empowering patients through critical paths. *Hospital Case Management* 1(1):1-2, Jan. 1993.

Hospital Case Management. Two community case managers save hospital a million dollars. *Hospital Case Management* 1(4):67, Apr. 1993a.

Hospital Case Management. Is case management the answer to coping with managed care? *Hospital Case Management* 1(6):104-6, 111, June 1993b.

Hospital Case Management. Pictorial pathways offer itineraries of hospital experience for patients. *Hospital Case Management* 1(8):141-42, Aug. 1993c.

Hospital Case Management. Positioning your program for success: the case management name game. *Hospital Case Management* 1(9):166-68, Sept. 1993d.

Hospital Case Management. Evaluating case management efforts beyond LOS data. *Hospital Case Management* 1(11):192, Nov. 1993e.

Hospital Case Management. Case management helps hospital prepare for capitated reimbursement. *Hospital Case Management* 2(2):26, 31-33, Feb. 1994.

Lamb, G. S., and Stempel, J. E. Nurse case management from the client's view: growing as an insider-expert. *Nursing Outlook* 42(1):7-13, Jan.-Feb. 1994.

Lumsdon, K., and Hagland, M. Mapping care. *Hospitals and Health Networks* 67(20):34-40, Oct. 20, 1993.

Riegel, B., Tomlinson, C., Weiss, M., Saks, N., Glancy, M., and Hanley, P. *Sharp Health-Care Manual for Clinical Mapping.* San Diego: Sharp HealthCare, Nov. 1993.

Zander, K. Focusing on patient outcome: case management in the 90s. *Dimensions of Critical Care Nursing* 11(3):127-29, May-June 1992.

Zander, K. *Managing Outcomes through Collaborative Care: The Application of Care Mapping and Case Management.* Chicago: American Hospital Publishing, 1995.

Zerull, L. Telephone interview with program director, case management, Winchester Medical Center, Winchester, VA, Feb. 12, 1994.

Chapter Four

How to Overcome Common Obstacles in Creating a Comprehensive Program

As emphasized throughout this book, planning and implementing a case management program is an ongoing process. In conceptualizing, developing, implementing, and modifying programs, organizations have experienced a number of common obstacles, including the following:

- Failure to grasp subtleties about the changing external environment
- Passive response to externally set standards
- Turf issues
- Inefficient reporting relationships
- Focus on tools instead of ultimate goals
- Inadequate information systems
- Leadership and accountability problems
- Physician issues (for example, conflicting financial incentives and potential loss of business)
- Policies and procedures that can impede case management
- Expectations of a quick fix or magical solution

Integrated financing and delivery systems with case management programs have experienced not only the obstacles listed, but also some systems-specific roadblocks. Those discussed in this book include:

- Moving from hospital-based to system-based case management
- Clinician relationships across organizations
- Failure to systematize technology
- Inadequate exchange of patient information
- Reimbursement incentives that hamper systemwide case management

This chapter describes these common problems and offers practical solutions and specific institutional examples.

Failure to Grasp Subtleties about the Changing External Environment

Many clinicians are overwhelmed by changes in their everyday work load. A common scenario is fewer inpatient beds, new staffing patterns, and anxiety over the redistribution of work. Most care givers do not take the time to think about subtleties of the changing *external* environment—new regulatory and licensing requirements, better informed consumers with more stringent demands, capitation, redistribution of risk, and so forth. Such subtleties, however, have created the necessity for case management.

The concept of capitation is a good example. The word is on everyone's lips these days, but it has different meanings for different people. To financial people, capitation implies less cash—paid earlier, to be sure, but bearing a new risk. To patient registration staff, capitation implies new responsibilities to ensure that services are provided only to enrollees covered by the capitation payment. To patient accounts staff, the capitation concept means less effort expended on collection. To the front-line staff who deliver patient care, the word may evoke images of the French Revolution.

The key point about capitation, as described in chapter 2, is that it shifts to providers the *opportunity* to assume responsibility for the *health* and care episode of a defined population. Most people miss the point completely and focus on capitation's likely impact on their own day-to-day responsibilities and bottom lines.

The key to explaining the implications of capitation, as well as other changes in the external environment, is to talk about the external environment *before* talking about a new case management program. Both group and individual sessions can provide discussion opportunities and set the stage for better acceptance of case management. Those whom it will affect need time to understand and process new concepts and implications for their roles in patient care.

Passive Response to Externally Set Standards

Provider assumption of risk and responsibility is a far cry from the health care industry's historic response to externally mandated rules and regulations. Traditionally, numerous regulatory and licensing bodies and diverse governmental levels laid out their expectations, and providers reacted by seeking to meet those standards. A common fear about national health reform is that yet more bureaucratic layers will result in even more onerous obligations from outside the health care system.

Good case management requires a *proactive* rather than a reactive approach, that is, setting *internal* standards for quality, cost-effectiveness, and continuity of patient care. The existence of internal standards does not mean that external ones are ignored, only that a certain level of expectation is set—and met—within an organization.

Turf Issues

Ideally, case management will become an organizational commitment, not a function taken over by one or two departments. In actuality, however, the ideal role for case management may be clouded by the historic turf issues that exist in all health care organizations.

Case management literature contains arguments advocating assignment of the responsibility to particular professions. The most common difference of opinion lies among nursing (patient services) and departments such as social service, discharge planning, or utilization review (Freeman 1992).

For example, one regional health system north of Boston, with 500-plus beds and providing a full spectrum of care including acute, rehabilitation, skilled nursing, and home care, created an elaborate and expensive system to introduce clinical paths and measure impact. It left untouched, however, the issue of which professionals were best suited to manage patient flow throughout the system. The acute care unit-based nurses, having a strong historic claim on "case management," prevailed over more objective suggestions to take the function away from direct care givers so that a manager/coordinator could move patients more efficiently through multiple levels of care.

Another New England system took a different approach. Instead of focusing on *who* should be the case manager, this system focused on *what* the case manager would do. When it became clear that the scope of responsibility would eventually extend beyond the walls of the acute care facility, direct care givers were ruled out as case managers and a new case management department was created by combining utilization review, discharge planning, and social service. The staff in these three departments were cross-trained; and, unlike the many part-time direct care givers, most were full-time employees who would be available to patients, families, and care givers around the clock.

Inefficient Reporting Relationships

Case management requires multidisciplinary cooperation, often among individuals and departments with a history of poor communication and, sometimes, competition. Providers with the most successful case management programs have taken an early and careful look at structure, making sure that it is consistent with the goals and scope of case management. For instance, in one community hospital with an effective program, the department reports directly to the COO. There is a dotted line between the case management department and the vice-president of managed care. The departments of utilization review, discharge planning, and social service have been combined into a new case management department, and the department head (recruited from the outside) has cross-trained all staff in the "art of case management." Prior to the development of case management, the utilization review, discharge planning, social service, and quality assurance staff reported to different vice-presidents—a strategy doomed to fail.

Focus on Tools Instead of Ultimate Goals

Sometimes care givers find it difficult to grasp the big picture in terms of case management. As mentioned in chapter 3, a common detour on the road to developing a workable program is an overemphasis on tools (such as clinical paths). In an article evaluating outcomes measurement in hospitals in a state mandating the use of a particular tool, Linder cautions that

> " . . . information technology is not deterministic. It does not structure an organization's behavior without the interest, initiative, and involvement of at least some influential members of the group. Organizational choice— taking responsibility for the decision to change—is an absolutely critical element in achieving results" (Linder 1992).

Thus, the purpose of doing case management—providing a smoother experience for patients as they move through various settings of care and tracking their resource utilization—needs to be stressed so that case managers use the tools appropriately.

Inadequate Information Systems

Information, as well as structure and reporting relationships, is a problem for many case management programs. Case managers need access to information on reimbursement denials, patient/family and physician satisfaction, and on physician practice patterns, so they can identify problems and seek solutions collaboratively.

If case management extends beyond the walls of an organization, case managers need even more data, that is, comprehensive information on what is happening to patients regardless of where care is rendered. Three facilities in which case managers have access to patient clinical and financial data in multiple settings are Sharp HealthCare and Friendly Hills in California and Carondelet St. Mary's in Arizona. As the Carondelet St. Mary's case management program expanded beyond the hospital walls, the nurse case managers responsible for seniors began to use laptop computers to facilitate access to information (Michaels 1992).

Leadership and Accountability Problems

Organizations most successful with their case management programs can identify a leader (the internal champion suggested in chapter 3) who understands the importance of case management and mobilizes the entire organization. This individual may not be the department head or senior executive to whom the department reports. He or she may be someone *outside* the operating loop, a visionary who understands the dynamics of the changing delivery system and encourages the organization to respond.

For example, at New England Medical Center (NEMC) in Boston, Massachusetts, the champion of nursing case management was an organizational development specialist and director of consultation services in the nursing department. With senior-level support, she implemented the program that became a model for many other organizations (Zander 1994).

At The Malden Hospital in Malden, Massachusetts, the vice-president for managed care played the role of champion, although the case management department reported to the chief operating officer.

At Winchester Medical Center in rural Virginia, the case management program got off to a slow start but was restructured so that a full-time director of case management assumed the role of champion or strategic thinker. The director reports directly to the vice-president for nursing, but the case managers, who are unit-based, report directly to the respective unit directors. The case management department director thus serves in a supportive role for her staff and can also focus on ongoing development (Zerull 1994).

At the integrated systems level, the vice-president, education, for Friendly Hills HealthCare Network in California was the organization's visionary. She hired a clinical nurse specialist to set up a pilot case management program, and when the pilot succeeded, the scope of case management expanded. At Sharp HealthCare, the vice-president for quality and mission is an important advocate for case management, as is the COO of one of the system's hospitals.

Physician Issues

Case management needs physician support, but many obstacles can stand in the way. They may range anywhere from conflicting financial incentives, to physicians' fear of losing business, to lack of physician leadership and vision, to disagreement between physician and hospital over how to manage care for end-of-life patients. These and other issues are discussed in the following subsections.

Conflicting Financial Incentives

Until such time as hospital and physician financial incentives are truly aligned, provider reimbursement is at cross purposes. Hospitals are accustomed to fixed payment, but many physicians continue to be paid on a fee-for-service basis. Thus physicians' financial incentive contrasts sharply with that of the hospital.

Dealing with conflicting incentives is difficult, but educating physicians about what lies ahead is an effective approach to circumventing this obstacle. Physicians who understand that fee-for-service will give way to capitation are more likely to cooperate in case management and other programs that, over time, will help them to manage their patients within a limited budget.

A special problem exists when physicians are paid on a salaried basis and may have no incentive for delivering care efficiently. Both tertiary and community providers have begun to address this issue by incorporating financial incentives for productivity and efficiency into physician compensation packages.

Potential Loss of Business

In one suburban metropolitan area where the competition among community hospitals was especially fierce, one hospital delayed its development of case management, fearing that the new program and the use of physician-specific information would be perceived as yet another challenge to their authority and cause physicians to take their patients elsewhere. The solution was to explain to physicians that physician-specific information on utilization would follow them, regardless of where they treated patients. That hospital could then address case management as a positive, not a negative, program.

Physician–Hospital Relations

Another obstacle to developing case management is the common physician perception that administrators are imposing case management on them, and that as care givers they have no role in program development. Brighton Medical Center in Portland, Maine, suggests that physician support can best be obtained through "a sell job, not a tell job" approach (*Hospital Case Management* 1993b). At Brighton, physicians drew their own conclusions about the value of case management—and they supported it.

An effective way to avoid physician misperception is to include them from the outset of the development of case management. Physicians actively involved in the assessment and learning phases will be more willing to support the program than the physicians whose involvement begins after decisions on program structure and operation have been made.

Physician Leadership and Vision

Lack of physician leadership and vision can be a major obstacle. One hospital with very clear administrative insight about the value of case management deliberately encouraged many physicians in different specialties to learn more about case management and to help design the program. The IPA president, a primary care physician, eventually asked the hospital to delegate to that organization physician responsibility for utilization management and quality assurance, including case management.

At Florida's HCA Tallahassee Community Hospital, a 180-bed facility, the hospital's public relations strategy with the physicians was successful, and the physicians were eager to accept the case managers as an extra set of hands to run interference (*Hospital Case Management* 1993b).

Service-Specific Input

Lack of service-specific input can impede physician support for case management. In many institutions, a limited number of physicians are involved in the utilization management/quality assurance/case management activities. Physicians who practice in a specialty not represented by the involved physician may prefer to have input from one of their own, a situation that easily can be addressed by case management. For example, obstetricians who are working to lower rates of Caesarean sections and to increase the frequency of vaginal births after C-section may prefer that their practices and outcomes be reviewed by another obstetrician.

Attitudes toward End-of-Life Patients

Case managers may encounter two physician obstacles related to end-of-life patients: (1) physician resistance to suggest noninstitutional alternatives for care, and (2) physician reluctance to discuss with patients and families the Do Not Resuscitate (DNR) option. A case manager who functions in a broker role rather than as a direct care giver may have the trust of physician, patient, and family, and be able to help each party work through their concerns. At both Friendly Hills HealthCare Network and Carondelet St. Mary's Hospital and Health Network, the case managers are expected to deal with end-of-life issues.

Policies and Procedures That Can Impede Case Management

Organizations that have introduced case management often refer to the program as their Pandora's box. Indeed, once the lid is opened, many other operational problems may come to light. Some of the operational policies and procedures that might impede case management are discussed in the following subsections.

Patient Registration and Booking

As case management programs evolve, case managers may find that their involvement with patients begins too late; that is, *after* an inappropriate admission has occurred or *after* an unnecessary procedure has been scheduled and performed. Some organizations have changed their admitting/scheduling procedures, and others have gone one step further and included case managers in the preadmission, booking, scheduling, and patient education processes.

At Baptist Memorial Hospital in Memphis, the case managers changed the timing of patient education from postoperative to preoperative care. Using diagnosis-specific critical paths (care paths) for guidance and teaching, they now begin patient education *prior to* admission. In some cases, the case managers go into the physician's office. For example, for lumbar laminectomies, patients are now educated when they are fully alert and able to ask questions about the expected course of treatment and recuperation. The level of education is a big improvement over the old system, where case managers approached patients *after* surgery and patients were too drowsy to absorb the message (*Hospital Case Management* 1993a).

Southwest General Hospital in Middleburg Heights, Ohio has a similar approach. The case management program integrates three components, inpatient, outpatient, and preadmission case management. The customer-service philosophy is the glue that holds all three components together (*Hospital Case Management* 1993c).

Emergency Department Admissions

Emergency department (ED) admissions can create two obstacles for case managers. If patients are admitted inappropriately through the ED, case manager involvement may come too late. Or, if care in the ED is rendered inefficiently, it can negatively affect the case manager's ability to manage the patient's subsequent care effectively.

A strategy against the first problem—inappropriate admission—is to use case management staff in the ED. For example, The Malden Hospital in Malden, Massachusetts, uses case managers to help with patients who clinically do not need hospitalization or ED treatment, but who indeed may need and appreciate their assistance in accessing other medical and nonmedical resources.

With respect to using case management in the ED to improve the efficiency of care, DeKalb Medical Center in Decatur, Georgia, has been particularly successful in treating chest pain patients. The case management concept has resulted in a newer and faster approach to ruling out myocardial infarction (*Hospital Case Management* 1993d).

Medical Education

The perception that residents escalate ordering patterns is hard to substantiate, because in many hospitals resident-specific data are not available from the information system. Hospitals take one of two approaches to encourage resident efficiency. Some focus only on the attending physicians, under the presumption that efficient attendings will convey the message. Others, like Stanford University Hospital, conduct resident education despite the difficulty of complicated rotation schedules.

Free Care, Financial Counseling, and Special Funds

A number of states have requirements regarding the availability of free care. Patients who avail themselves of such programs may have expectations that are inconsistent with the recommendations of the case manager and the physician. Particularly if inpatient care is "free" but outpatient care is not, a patient may have a strong incentive to extend the length of stay. Similarly, if inpatient acute care is "free" but nursing home care requires the patient to pay, the patient and family may try to prolong the acute stay.

An effective way to deal with the free care issue is to be very clear up front about the content and duration of the treatment plan, covering both the inpatient and the aftercare components. If only part of the care will be free, the issue of what comes next and who will pay can be dealt with as early as possible.

A creative approach to patients with inadequate resources was developed by Tampa General Hospital in 1987. Its Safe Ways for Alternative Treatment (SWAT) program saved over $7.57 million in nonreimbursable days over four years by spending $573,135 (*Hospital Peer Review* 1992).

The SWAT program uses an interdisciplinary team to assess patient need. Patients who can be discharged safely to a lower level of care, but who do not have the resources to cover the cost of necessary continuing care, are identified. If the cost of caring for the patient in the acute environment is much greater than the cost of continuing care at a lower level, the hospital assists in purchasing needed items such as home infusion treatment, durable medical equipment, supplies, guardianship services, and transportation. Funds for the program are included in the hospital's operating budget.

Expectations of a Quick Fix or Magical Solution

There is no one 'right' way to develop case management. More than one organization has failed to come up with an effective program because it sought a quick-and-dirty approach—borrowing someone else's solution. There is no substitute for process, and for the ongoing discussion that needs to take place about goals, structure, strengths and weaknesses, resources, and suitability for a changing delivery system.

The case management program at Carondelet St. Mary's Hospital and Health Center in Tucson, Arizona, described in detail in chapter 7, exemplifies the way a program may evolve over time. The nurse case management program began in 1985 with hospitalized patients, but as its value in health promotion and health maintenance became clear, it expanded to other populations, including seniors and young pregnant women with substance abuse problems (Michaels 1992). The "beyond-the-walls" approach to case management has become a model for other programs throughout the country, and nurse case management services are now available to people with chronic illness, patients recovering from acute illness who need temporary help, and terminally ill patients.

Case management at New England Medical Center (NEMC) is another example of an evolutionary approach. The Center's original case management program focused on the role of the nurse case manager and on the measurement of variance from expected protocol. The program was truly visionary in that DRG-based reimbursement had not yet come to Massachusetts (Grossman 1994; Etheredge 1994).

Payer demands and new methods of reimbursement, along with a new attention to customer demands and to patient-centered care, have affected NEMC in the 1990s. Nursing case management has been replaced by a multidisciplinary practice pattern initiative program that emphasizes delivery of high-quality, cost-effective care as efficiently as possible, while meeting the needs of the patient—regardless of where he or she is receiving care. Physicians are more involved now, and there is more interest in the measurement and improvement of outcomes to complement the focus on best practices and variances from expected protocol (Etheredge 1994).

At Stanford University Hospital in Stanford, California, the initial focus of case management was on specific service lines. (Chapter 1 describes the success of case management for urology and oncology inpatients, highlighting the effectiveness of the case manager/social service worker team.) Stanford's case management program has evolved over time and now extends beyond the inpatient focus into the community and into the faculty clinics (Day 1994). The concept of a community case manager was developed when the hospital began participating in a capitated HMO Medicare risk contract. When Medicare clients sign up for the plan and select a primary care physician, the medical group partner administers a risk assessment questionnaire containing 20 variables. The physician assistants who work with the physician groups and the hospital's community nurse case managers review the results. If an enrollee qualifies as "high risk," the community case manager establishes and maintains contact in order to coordinate the use of health care resources.

Extension of case management into Stanford's faculty clinics was done selectively, and there are now ambulatory case managers in the pain, obstetrics/gynecology, gynecology/oncology, and bone marrow transplant clinics. The ambulatory case manager for obstetrics/gynecology works closely with the inpatient case manager if the patient is hospitalized. The other ambulatory case managers coordinate both outpatient and inpatient care if the patient is admitted.

As Stanford has moved toward an integrated delivery system, case management has been shifted from its initial reporting relationship in patient services into the new quality support department. The new department reports directly to the chief medical officer (Day 1994).

Systems-Specific Obstacles

Although integrated systems may create a formal and legally sanctioned continuum of care, *clinical integration* of care may be lacking (Conrad 1993). Case management, one of several ways to manage patients in a systems context, may not work at all if other issues are not addressed simultaneously. Some of these issues—moving from hospital-based to systems-based case management, clinician relationships across organizations, failure to systemize technology, inadequate exchange of patient information, reimbursement incentives that hamper systemwide case management—are summarized briefly in the following subsections.

Moving from Hospital-Based to System-Based Case Management

In a number of integrated financing and delivery systems, case management was established within one of the system components—usually an acute or tertiary hospital—before the system began to focus on case management across the continuum of care. Two examples are Sharp HealthCare (chapter 8) and Lutheran General (chapter 9). In these situations, the challenge is not to undo what has been accomplished, but to build on it in an appropriate way in the larger systems context.

Clinician Relationships across Organizations

Systems need to address many issues relating to clinician relationships across organizations. For example, if admitting or treatment privileges are restricted to certain parts of the system, physicians and other professionals may be discouraged from using the total array of available resources. Also, lack of consensus on appropriate patterns of care, patient outcomes, and on tools such as practice guidelines and protocols can hinder patient-focused case management. Finally, clinicians in different settings who do not know each other personally and who do not share philosophies of patient care are less likely to provide coordinated care than those who do. Attention to these issues can make a big difference in efficiently provided patient care in multiple settings.

Failure to Systematize Technology

As systems develop, they begin to deal with the use of technologies in their different components. Without clinical coordination of these technologies, however, case managers may encounter system inconsistencies that affect how they do their job. For example, different components of a system that is legally but not clinically integrated may give rise to repeat of costly diagnostic tests as patients move from point to point. Case management cannot solve the problem of resource duplication, but it can highlight problems.

Inadequate Exchange of Patient Information

Clinical integration of care is highly dependent on information systems. The computerized medical record (CPR) is the tool that will enable systems to capture patient-specific information over time, and to organize and distribute it to appropriate users. Until the CPR is in place, however, case managers must struggle with different sources of information.

Reimbursement Incentives That Hamper Systemwide Case Management

Systems expand in stages, and the cart sometimes gets ahead of the horse. With respect to reimbursement for care, the ultimate system goal is to be able to accept and distribute a lump sum among the different providers of care, and to manage the risk associated with receipt of the funds.

When systems are in their early growth stages, however, reimbursement may be fragmented, and parts of the system may still be rewarded for providing more rather than less care. Case management in such an environment is a challenge, to say the least.

References and Bibliography

Certification for Case Management. Rolling Meadows, IL, Certification of Insurance Rehabilitation Specialist Commission, Sept. 1992.

Conrad, D. A. Coordinating patient care services in regional health systems: the challenge of clinical integration. *Journal of the Foundation of the ACHE,* 38(4):491–508, Winter 1993.

Day, C. Telephone interviews with director of social services and utilization management, Stanford University Hospital, Stanford, CA, Apr. 18, 25, and Sept. 26, 1994.

Etheredge, M. L. S. Telephone interview with director of nursing education, New England Medical Center, Boston, MA, Mar. 18, 1994.

Freeman, E. Who is better prepared to fill the role of case manager? Nurses or social workers? *JANAC* 3(2):36–37, Apr.–June 1992.

Grossman, J. H. Interview with president, New England Medical Center, Boston, MA, Jan. 6, 1994.

Hospital Case Management. Tennessee hospital includes advance directive choices on critical path. *Hospital Case Management* 1(1):3, Jan. 1993a.

Hospital Case Management. How to win physician support for hospital case management programs. *Hospital Case Management* 1(2):21–23, Feb. 1993b.

Hospital Case Management. Integrated case management: model combines cost containment and quality. *Hospital Case Management* 1(6):114, June 1993c.

Hospital Case Management. The fast path: case management enters the emergency department. *Hospital Case Management* 1(11):200–202, Nov. 1993d.

Hospital Peer Review 17(4):49–52, Apr. 1992.

Linder, J. C. Outcomes measurement in hospitals: can the system change the organization? *Hospitals and Health Services Administration* 37(2):160, Summer 1992.

Michaels, C. Carondelet St. Mary's nursing enterprise. *Nursing Administration* 27(3):77–85, Mar. 1992.

Zander, K. Interview in Boston with principal and co-owner, The Center for Case Management, Natick, MA, Mar. 29, 1994.

Zerull, L. Telephone interview with program director, case management, Winchester Medical Center, Winchester, VA, Feb. 12, 1994.

Chapter Five

Creation of a Case Management Program at The Malden Hospital

This chapter describes the conceptualization and set-up of case management at The Malden Hospital, in Malden, Massachusetts. The example is included in the book for two reasons. First, it demonstrates that the development of case management is a process, not an act. The efforts of the hospital and physicians *before* establishing a program contributed to the ultimate outcome. Second, the example illustrates the importance of involving a multidisciplinary group of clinical and nonclinical health care professionals.

The chapter is divided into the following main sections:

- Description of case management and the outcome
- Background
- The players
- The problems
- Positive forces for change
- Important points

Description of Case Management and the Outcome

Case management at The Malden Hospital was conceptualized early in 1992 and implemented later that year. Eighteen months after the program was launched, the hospital and physicians had accomplished the following:

- Case management had become an organizational priority for managing patient care, not just a function taken over by one or two departments.
- A new case management department had been set up and reported to the executive vice-president/chief operating officer. Its activities and positive approach to patient problem solving had informally extended beyond the acute

Information for this chapter was obtained through the author's personal experience and from the director of case management at The Malden Hospital, Evelyn M. Soldano, R.N., M.A., C.C.M.

79

inpatient setting into office-based practices, ambulatory clinics, emergency department, home care, long-term care, and other settings. (See figure 5-1.)
- Five case managers had been cross-trained in utilization review and discharge planning and assigned to work with individual physicians/groups.
- Social service staff in the case management department provided consultation services to specific categories of high-risk inpatients and had extended case management activities into areas other than the inpatient setting.
- Physicians in the hospital's independent practice association (IPA) had formally assumed responsibility for the medical component of the utilization management and quality assurance activities. Their involvement enhanced the case managers' ability to influence physician behavior.
- Case management had had a measurable impact in terms of staff, patient, and family satisfaction; quality improvement; increased communication/

Figure 5-1. Long-Range Application of Case Management, North Suburban Health Systems, Inc.

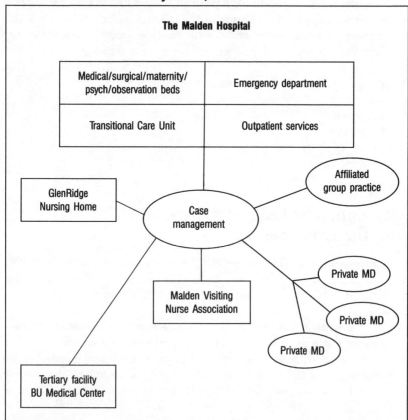

Source: Reprinted, with permission, from The Malden Hospital, Malden, MA, 1994.

collaboration; financial indicators (that is, denial of payment, elimination of administratively necessary days, and reduction in average charges per Medicare case).

* The hospital and physicians felt confident about their ability to manage patient care and actively sought out risk-based arrangements with managed care plans.

To achieve these outcomes, the hospital and physicians took the following 10 steps:

1. Acknowledged the existence of problems with the continuity of patient care and physician input into hospital utilization management and quality assurance activities
2. Reached a common understanding of the generic concept of case management and agreed on the appropriate application of it at The Malden Hospital
3. Agreed on the short-term and long-term goals of case management
4. Decided on appropriate reporting relationships and staffing needs
5. Hired a director of case management
6. Cross-trained staff from the utilization review, discharge planning, and social service departments
7. Involved physicians in the development, implementation, and ongoing evolution of the case management program
8. Developed measures to monitor the impact of the case management program
9. Explored the use of tools to facilitate case management
10. Continued on an ongoing basis to search for new ways in which case management could improve patient care

The hospital and its physicians were satisfied with their progress to date and expected that their case management program would continue to evolve. At least the following future challenges lay before them: continuation of collaborative efforts between clinical and financial staff; development of tools to facilitate case management (for example, practice guidelines, outcomes measurement); development of information on case management into educational and informational tools for patients, families, and payers; formal expansion of case management beyond the acute inpatient setting.

Background

The Malden Hospital is a 200-bed facility in Malden, Massachusetts, a New England community with a population of 52,000 residents. The primary service area population is 181,800. The hospital is easily accessible to Boston by public transportation and is within 10 minutes' driving distance of five other community hospitals.

As part of a community-based system of care, the hospital is a subsidiary of North Suburban Health Systems, Inc. Other North Suburban subsidiaries are GlenRidge Nursing Home, a day care center, and a management service organization. Malden's Visiting Nurse Association (VNA), once a holding company subsidiary, is now a hospital department. As a teaching affiliate of a major metropolitan hospital, the system admitted most patients requiring tertiary care to that institution.

At the time that The Malden Hospital began its discussions about the importance of case management, it was not involved in network discussions with other community and tertiary providers. By 1994, however, the hospital and physicians were actively engaged in discussions with a tertiary facility, other community hospitals, and a major insurer.

As a full-service community hospital, Malden provides a broad spectrum of inpatient and ambulatory services. The inpatient services are medical/surgical, maternity, psychiatric, and transitional care. As the market continues to demand cost-effective and efficiently delivered care of the highest quality, the hospital has been flexible in converting beds to alternative uses. Furthermore, the facility is experiencing a continuing shift from inpatient to outpatient business and is encouraging, not resisting, that change.

The Malden Hospital is well along with a major project, jointly sponsored by the city government, to assess community needs and respond appropriately. Because the service area has large numbers of elderly and Asian residents, the hospital needs to be able to understand and respond to the specific needs of these groups.

Primary care is a priority, and the hospital has begun an ambitious long-term program that includes the development of a Malden-based family practice residency program. It also includes the acquisition of primary care practices in the surrounding service area.

Malden physicians established an IPA early in 1992 and membership grew quickly to 150 physicians in all specialties. Although the IPA has been in existence for a relatively short time, its officers and board quickly grasped the importance of physician–hospital joint efforts and physician responsibility for care management. The IPA has taken the initiative in developing a risk-sharing arrangement with an HMO that involved selection of some but not all of the primary care physicians as participants.

Before the formal introduction of case management, The Malden Hospital had a case management task force, a group chaired by the executive vice-president/chief operating officer to look at the potential for the development of such a program. Task force members included the executive vice-president, three hospital vice-presidents (patient services, planning, and general services), and staff from utilization review, discharge planning, social service, quality assurance, and home care. Two physicians, a medical specialist and an internist who was medical director of quality assurance/utilization review, were part of the group.

Two factors stimulated The Malden Hospital's serious interest in developing a formal case management program. One was the arrival of a new vice-president for managed care, and the other was the sudden and rapid change in the health care environment. It was clear that payers would pay less, that providers would be forced to accept increased risk, and that the most successful providers would be those that knew how to move patients through a continuum of care with maximum efficiency. In a state with over 35 percent managed care penetration, providers had a long and hard way to go. Conceptually, case management made sense.

The Players

At The Malden Hospital, people and personalities made a difference in case management. Prior to the formal development of a case management program, the key person had been the executive vice-president/chief operating officer (EVP/COO), who chaired the hospital's case management task force. The EVP/COO was responsible for day-to-day hospital operations and had a general understanding of case management. Another important player had been the medical director for utilization review and quality assurance, an internist who had been in his position for 15 years.

The director of utilization review, the third key person, had been a discharge planner for most of her career and was uncomfortable in the supervisory aspects of her role as department head. The social service department, including discharge planning, reported to her. Utilization review reported to the vice-president for general services, as did the director of quality assurance. A partial organization chart for The Malden Hospital prior to implementation of a formal case management program is shown in figure 5-2.

The introduction and implementation of case management introduced a new cast of characters. Among them were the new vice-president, managed care; the director of case management; the first president of Malden's IPA, who later became IPA medical director; and the second IPA president.

The vice-president, managed care, was the first person to hold that position. She was responsible for the strategic and operational aspects of managed care and reported directly to the hospital's president. Acutely aware of the fierce competition among community hospitals in Malden's service area, she nevertheless believed that case management could distinguish the hospital from its competitors and enhance its "managed care readiness"—an idea strongly supported by the president.

The EVP/COO and vice-president, managed care, jointly hired Malden's first director of case management—an R.N. with master's-level training. She had prior case management experience in a large insurance company and had also worked in discharge planning in a community hospital.

**Figure 5-2. Organizational Chart Prior to Case Management,
The Malden Hospital**

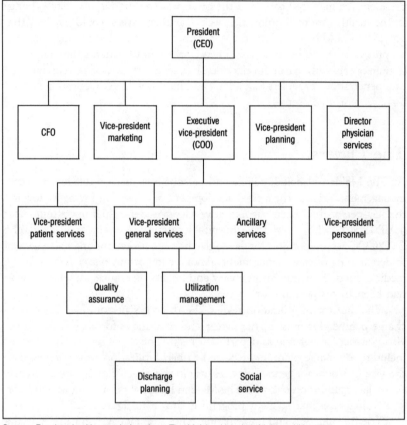

Source: Reprinted, with permission, from The Malden Hospital, Malden, MA, 1994.

The internist who was the first IPA president was strongly committed to physician involvement in utilization management and quality improvement. Upon ultimately assuming the role of IPA medical director, he was succeeded as IPA president by a family practitioner.

Some Problems and Solutions

Once the hospital had identified case management as a potential managed care strategy, a number of problems surfaced. Chief among them were an ambiguous definition of case management; inadequate motivation; physician issues; financial issues; reporting relationships; and measurement issues. These problems are discussed in more detail in the following subsections.

Ambiguous Definition of Case Management

Although The Malden Hospital had a case management task force, members of the group did not share an understanding of the concept's basic definition or potential application in their own institution/system. In general, each task force member held a discipline-specific notion of the meaning of the term *case management*. Most still thought of it as something that might be done *to* patients by external agencies or health plans; they did not appreciate the opportunity presented to them to develop an internally driven case management program.

The task force was confused about the activities of utilization management, discharge planning, social service, and quality improvement, and about the way in which case management could potentially link them together. It also did not understand the relationship between the *process* of case management and its *tools* (for example, clinical practice guidelines and protocols) for making the process work.

The solution: Once the hospital decided to fully explore the development of case management, it engaged an outside consultant to explain the concept to the seven-person senior management group and then to a reconstituted and expanded case management work group. The expanded group included many of the original task force members and additional physicians. The consultant had experience in other parts of the country. As an outsider, she was able to explain the generic meaning of case management as a patient-focused approach.

Inadequate Motivation

Although senior managers at Malden had a good understanding of changes in the external environment that required a new provider mind-set, some of the middle managers and other professionals had partial or no information. Their vocabulary excluded the terms *vertical integration, capitation, management of risk,* and *low-cost/high-quality services.* The rapidly changing role of the acute hospital was not well understood.

The hospital and physicians had access to, but did not make good use of, existing data that compared its performance with that of competing institutions and that also compared individual practice patterns. Without hard data, there was little incentive to look for improvement.

The solution: To clarify important concepts and to explain to senior managers, physicians, and other professionals what the outside world knew about The Malden Hospital and physicians, the vice-president, managed care, presented several educational sessions on the managed care environment. She also initiated a data collection project directed toward quantifying and interpreting comparative hospital and physician information.

Physician Issues

Three physician-specific issues hindered the development of case management. These were historic lack of physician participation in hospital decision making;

conflicting physician/hospital financial incentives; and inadequate understanding of state-of-the-art developments (for example, standard treatment protocols, benchmarks, and clinical practice guidelines).

Historically, The Malden Hospital had not included physicians in its planning process. Many physicians retained a basic mistrust of the hospital's administration, blaming the president for the changes in medical practice that were affecting all Massachusetts physicians. Case management could not succeed, however, without mutual trust and a multidisciplinary effort.

In Massachusetts, over 35 percent of the population was enrolled in managed care plans. Unlike California and Minnesota, however, Massachusetts HMOs and PPOs were not as far along with provider risk sharing. Most plans had inconsistent financial incentives, motivating hospitals to reduce the inpatient length of stay but retaining physician incentives to extend the provision of inpatient care. Unless the reimbursement incentives were aligned, physicians and hospitals would lack a common financial incentive to alter behavior.

The hospital's physicians participated in many managed care plans, but they lacked sophisticated understanding of state-of-the-art developments in health care. For example, most perceived capitation as a different method of payment but did not comprehend the responsibility aspect of capitation (that is, the obligation to keep patients healthy and out of the health care system). Similarly, most physicians did not understand the relationship between the case management process and some of the tools that would help it work.

The solution: The process of learning about case management and developing a program at The Malden Hospital was a multidisciplinary effort, involving physicians as well as administrators and clinicians. The physicians helped make decisions on program design—a real change from their usual experience of hearing about a new program after the hospital had developed it unilaterally.

The financial incentive issue was difficult, and the hospital took an indirect approach. Its strategy of physician practice acquisition helped align the financial incentives of some of the physicians and the hospital; but at the time case management was developing, most physicians were still in private practice. By creating user-friendly comparative data, The Malden Hospital introduced a somewhat different incentive to its physicians—competition amongst themselves. For example, each chief of service had access to DRG-specific information comparing resource utilization by different physicians. The chiefs worked with their services to identify problem areas and improve the consistency with which care was delivered. Despite the mixed hospital/physician reimbursement incentives, the physician-specific data had the desired effect. Physician education for the entire medical staff addressed the problem of lack of familiarity with important new concepts. For example, the medical director of a large corporation talked about corporate interest in quality and provider selectivity. A state medical society representative introduced the use of practice guidelines, and a physician from a successful HMO in a distant part of the state talked about that plan's quality activities.

Financial Issues

Although the case management department anticipated differences of opinion with insurance company representatives, the director and her staff also encountered a number of financial issues within the hospital. For example, case managers needed information from patient accounts on denied reimbursement so that they could identify problems and take corrective action. Patient accounts initially had no such information system in place but eventually developed one.

A second financial issue was free care. All Massachusetts hospitals had a legal obligation to fund free care for patients who could not afford to pay. As a result, the case managers often encountered situations where they and the physician recommended discharge, but patients preferred to remain in the hospital.

The solution: Case management and patient accounts developed a good working relationship over time. Once case management had information on denials for both inpatient care, and ultimately for emergency department and outpatient care, the case management staff took a leadership role in working with other clinicians to reduce the number and amount of denied payments.

With respect to the free care issue, investigation revealed that The Malden Hospital had gone beyond its legal obligation of informing patients about free care. The process for distributing patient information subsequently was reviewed and changed.

Reporting Relationships

As the hospital's case management work group talked through case management, it became clear that some of the reporting relationships no longer made sense. Historically, those most involved in the movement of patients through the hospital and into holding company subsidiaries reported to the vice-president, general services. Such staff received minimal guidance on new developments in the management and coordination of patient care. Also, social service, including discharge planning, reported to the director of utilization review, who preferred to be back in the trenches doing discharge planning and did not offer good direction. Existing reporting relationships did not facilitate new ideas.

The solution: In any organization, moving people around is sensitive. The Malden Hospital instructed the outside consultant to put heavy emphasis on the structure most appropriate for the patient. Discussions about case management did not become turf battles. The voluntary resignation of the director of utilization review was timely and offered an opportunity for realignment. Figure 5-3 is a partial organization chart for the hospital following the development of case management.

Figure 5-3. Organizational Chart Subsequent to Case Management, The Malden Hospital

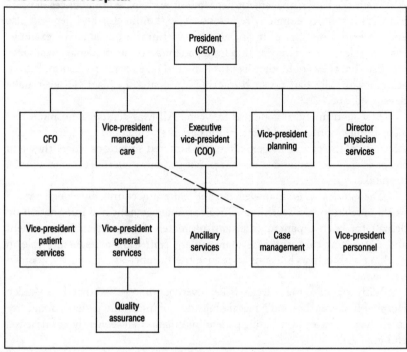

Source: Reprinted, with permission, from The Malden Hospital, Malden, MA, 1994.

Data Measurement Issues

Although the vice-president, managed care, initiated a project to produce comparative data, the available information had many flaws. For example, the facility had no cost accounting system, so that the comparative information was charge-based. Also, the available information was not adjusted for severity.

A second measurement issue was ongoing responsibility for maintaining and using the data base. The initial data project had been done with outside assistance, and the hospital was uncertain how to integrate the measurement of hospital and physician performance into its ongoing quality measurement activities.

The solution: Malden used its quality council, representing hospital staff, physicians, and board, to give shape and guidance to the ongoing efforts to collect and use data for quality improvement, including case management.

Positive Forces for Change

Despite the problems just described, The Malden Hospital and its physicians developed, implemented, and have continued to enhance case management in a way that meets their needs and budget. Factors that contribute to the program's success are:

- Support from top levels of the organization
- Cooperative relationship among the staff and line senior managers
- Use of the vice-president, managed care, as the case management internal visionary and champion
- Use of outside consultants
- Staff turnover
- Extraordinary cooperation from patient services
- Physician involvement in the decision process
- Addressing hospital problems prior to physician practice issues

The factors are discussed in more detail in the following subsections.

Support from Top Levels of the Organization

The Malden Hospital president was receptive to the case management concept from the outset. He encouraged the managed care vice-president and EVP/COO to work jointly, and he supported a multidisciplinary approach to decision making and implementation.

Cooperative Relationship among Staff and Line Senior Managers

Although the case management director has jokingly described herself as the "filling in a sandwich," she benefited from the involvement of two vice-presidents in her department's activity. The EVP/COO offered ongoing guidance on operational problems. Because Patient Services reported to him, he was in a good position to facilitate interdepartmental coordination. The managed care vice-president sat outside the operating loop and offered ideas on new program development and measurement. The working relationship between the two senior managers was cooperative and supportive to case management.

Use of an Internal Case Management Champion

As the in-house expert on the theory and concept of case management, the vice-president, managed care, offered an unusual resource. She did not deal with day-to-day problems with staff or with patients/families but focused on program development and marketing.

Both the vice-president, managed care, and the case management director were constantly on the lookout for successful programs in other parts of the country. At the same time that Malden was developing its program, the vice-president, managed care, was writing this book on case management, and she had access to information about case management programs in both single organizations and integrated financing and delivery systems. Much of what she learned was applied at The Malden Hospital.

Use of Outside Consultants

The Malden Hospital made good use of two outside consultants. The first explained the concept of case management to various groups, interviewed physicians and staff on an individual basis, and suggested structure and staffing for case management that were specific to the hospital's particular situation. She did not use a cookbook approach to case management but customized her recommendations to fit the client.

The second consultant assisted with managed care long-range planning and data. His good working relationship with physicians helped educate them and encouraged the IPA leadership to take a more assertive role in utilization management and quality assurance activities.

Staff Turnover

The voluntary retirement of the director of utilization review coincided with the development of case management and facilitated reorganization of the utilization review, discharge planning, and social service departments.

Extraordinary Cooperation from Patient Services

In setting up its case management program, Malden avoided a problem commonly encountered in acute care hospitals—the insistence of patient services that case management be a nursing division function, regardless of the logic of this approach. The Malden case managers were nurses by training, but they did not report to the nursing division. The inpatient nurse staffing at the hospital did not lend itself to case management by nurses as direct care givers. Many of the nurses worked part-time, and given the hospital's desire to assign one case manager to each physician to be available around the clock, the arrangement would not work. Also, as the case management work group talked about the role of the case managers and of potentially extending the process beyond the acute care setting, it became clear that at Malden, professionals other than nurses as direct care givers were better suited to assume responsibility for case management.

Over time, the relationship between the case management department and patient services took an interesting twist. The assignment of one case manager to each physician was working well, and the physicians liked the easy access to a single individual for information about all of their patients. Patient services offered to test a parallel approach and to divide the direct care givers into teams to work with physicians and case managers. Documentation by nurses and case managers would be coordinated and simplified so that physicians could find the information they needed in one place.

Physician Involvement in Program Development

Physician involvement in the development of case management was present at the outset and improved over time. The hospital included both formal and informal leaders of the medical staff and IPA in the planning and implementation processes so that physicians would feel comfortable with the new program.

The strategy succeeded. Much to the hospital's delight, the IPA developed the physician component for case management. Guided by the IPA president and medical director, a group of four primary care physicians worked closely with the case management and quality assurance staffs.

Addressing Hospital Problems Prior to Physician Practice Issues

The Malden Hospital knew at the outset that physician support for case management was important, and the assignment of case managers to individual physicians occurred within two months after the director was hired. With respect to daily physician involvement in managing care, however, the hospital took the time to work through its own staffing issues before it addressed physician practice patterns.

Important Points

Following are eight guidelines offered as a result of the case management experience at The Malden Hospital. Organizations seeking to implement case management can use them for direction as they develop customized programs that best meet their needs.

- Do not assume that everyone understands the environment and accepts the rationale for case management. Explain it over and over again.
- Clearly explain the organization-specific definition of case management, specifying boundaries of responsibility, scope of authority, direct care giver/coordinator of care, relationship of tools to process, and so on.
- Be sure senior managers are committed to case management.
- Make case management an organizational activity, not a departmental approach.
- Expect a lengthy process, not quick results.
- Identify a champion or visionary who may not have day-to-day operational responsibility for case management.
- Do not reinvent the wheel; use existing resources to find out what others have done.
- Case management is never finished; instead, it is evolutionary, keeping abreast of the rapidly changing health care environment.

The Integrated Case Management Network at Friendly Hills HealthCare Network

Friendly Hills HealthCare, in La Habra, California, is an integrated provider system based around a large, multispecialty group practice. Unlike other integrated systems that grow out of hospitals, the focal point is ambulatory care. In fact, the word *discharge* is not a part of the Friendly Hills vocabulary—enrollees experience "transition" from service point to service point. (The Friendly Hills continuum of care is shown in figure 6-1.) Both clinical nurse specialists and geriatric nurse practitioners provide case management. This chapter describes the program, highlighting the role of the geriatric case manager. It is divided into the following key sections:

- Background
- Case management network goal, design, and target population
- Staffing issues (responsibilities, skills, training)
- Geriatric case management
- Important points

Background

The Friendly Hills system is responsible for 100,000 prepaid patients, including 15,000 seniors, and is at full risk for system enrollees. Ninety-five percent of its revenue is derived from 26 fully capitated managed care contracts. There are 150 providers at eleven office sites and one 297-bed hospital.

In the spring of 1994, the medical center affiliate of Friendly Hills, Loma Linda University Medical Center, announced plans to join with Adventist Health System/West to form the large regional system Pacific Integrated Healthcare (PIH). When the framework for the Friendly Hills delivery system was developed, there were no systems in place to manage and coordinate patient care across the continuum. A new vice-president, education, recruited from outside

Information for the chapter was provided by Nancy Brown, R.N. (vice-president, education); Alison Jacoby, R.N., M.S.N. (cardiopulmonary clinical nurse); and Lynn Mumaw, R.N., M.S.N. (geriatric nurse practitioner).

Figure 6-1.   Continuum of Care, Friendly Hills HealthCare Network

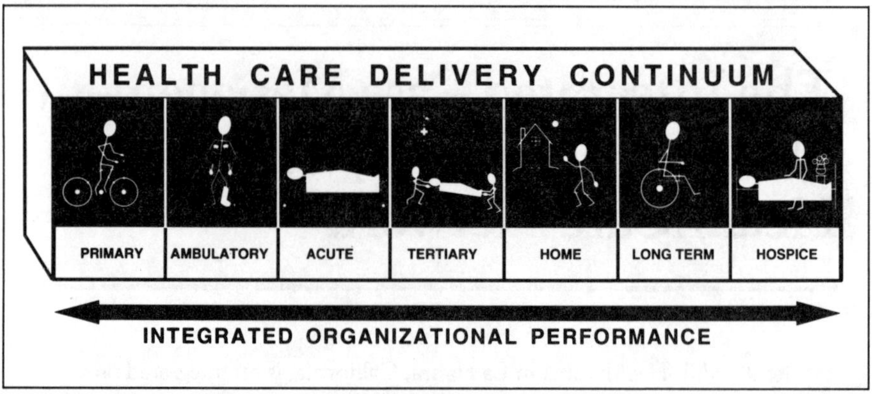

Source: Reprinted, with permission, from *Beyond Strategy: Operational Issues in a Capitated Health Care System*. La Habra, CA: Friendly Hills HealthCare Network, 1994.

the organization, addressed this need by developing a network to case manage patients seen at multiple access points by more than one provider.

In contrast to organizations that encourage multidisciplinary input to the development of case management and that take a long time for conceptualization, Friendly Hills introduced the concept quietly. Geriatric nurse practitioners were already working within the system, and a clinical nurse specialist (CNS) was hired to head up the case management network. The network head also carries her own case load. Initially case management had no budget. But once the program had succeeded and expanded, it became a separate line item.

Case Management Network Goal, Design, and Target Population

The goal of the Friendly Hills case management network is to apply a case management process in order to achieve four key objectives. These are to optimize the patient's functional and self-care capabilities, prevent complications, facilitate system access to services and communication with the health care team, and coordinate appropriate utilization of resources.

Friendly Hills enrollees are the focal point of both the delivery system and case management. The network of case managers includes both clinical nurse specialists and geriatric nurse practitioners. Each CNS is responsible for a case load within a defined area of expertise (for example, cardiovascular, oncology, maternal-child, nephrology). Referrals come from ambulatory sites or elsewhere in the Friendly Hills system when providers perceive that enrollees have potential problems or may be among a high-risk population.

In developing the case management network, Friendly Hills identified those clinical areas where enrollees are at the highest risk. Within each specialty, the

CNS has the challenge of developing "case load criteria" to determine the appropriate targets for case management.

Examples of criteria used to define the target population for case management are patients who fall into the following categories:

- Seen in the emergency department for medical care for the same diagnosis more than two or three times per month
- Admitted three or more times per year for the same diagnosis
- Referred to tertiary care
- Discharged on oxygen, ventilators, or with home health services
- Shown to require extended care placement

When justification for inclusion in the case management case load no longer exists, care continues without the direct involvement of the case manager.

The case managers in all specialty areas have strong working relationships with the hospital's utilization management department and with managed care. (The managed care department handles business operations, claims, and benefits.)

Staffing Issues

The case managers are responsible for both coordination of care and for the financial impact of resource utilization. To do their jobs, they need a broad set of skills.

Regardless of specialty, all case managers need advanced degrees and knowledge of the following: health care systems, operations, patient/family dynamics, and communication and problem-solving skills. Each specialist performs a different role for her target population and therefore needs specialty-specific knowledge of care givers and resources. For example, the CNS for cardiovascular services has strong working relationships with cardiologists, with cardiac surgeons, and with cardiac rehabilitation programs. The CNS for oncology deals with a completely different cast of characters and resources.

Friendly Hills did not look to staff already in the system to perform the case management role. Rather, it recruited from outside, looking for CNSs with clinical expertise in specialty areas. The clinical nurse specialists and the geriatric nurse practitioners are all master's prepared. Friendly Hills' own staff—administrative, medical, financial—taught the case managers some of the non-clinical skills they needed.

Geriatric Case Management

There are five geriatric nurse practitioner case managers at Friendly Hills. Each one focuses on a broad spectrum of needs and services of the elderly population, including those of nursing home patients who qualify as high risk. The case managers coordinate care by working closely with both physicians in the family practice department and hospital utilization management staff. Figure 6-2 outlines a case management case study for a geriatric CABG patient, and figure 6-3 (p. 98) shows a CABG clinical path.

The geriatric case managers may intervene at different points in the continuum of care. For example, they may talk with patients and families *before* the decision to admit to a nursing home has been made. At the point of admission, they may raise the issue of a do not resuscitate (DNR) order, so that patients and families understand their options. After nursing home admission, the case managers visit with patients regularly and also make sure that families are kept well informed about patient care.

Figure 6-2. CABG Case Management Case Study, Friendly Hills HealthCare Network

---

Background

A. H. is a 71-year-old male with a history of coronary artery disease. He has been stable, managed with medication since his first onset of symptoms five years ago. He now presents with a one-month history of increasing episodes of angina with mild exertion. A recent treadmill stress test was positive for isonemia, and cardiac catheterization showed severe LAD and RCA disease. Friendly Hills (FHHN) cardiologists determined the patient to be a probable candidate for open-heart surgery and referred him to Loma Linda University Medical Center (LLUMC) for cardiac surgery evaluation.

Patient Cardiac Risk Factors

- Ten-year history of hypertension controlled with medication
- Cholesterol level
- Family history: father died of MI at age 60, brother died of MI at age 62
- Quit smoking one year ago (smoked one pack per day for 25 years)
- No history of diabetes

Social

Married for 38 years, patient lives with his wife who is disabled with COPD and requires continuous home oxygen. He has two grown children who are both married and live out of state. A retired engineer, he has very few hobbies, friends, or outside interests due to his primary role as care giver to his wife.

Exercise 1: At this point in time, locate where the patient and his wife are accessing the system on the continuum of care. Discuss the goals for the patient and his wife at the point on the continuum. What barriers might be anticipated that would prevent the patient from moving along the continuum? Discuss the tools and/or resources that might be mobilized to assist moving the patient along the continuum.

The patient has a 3V CABG at LLUMC and is discharged home in six days with no complications. Both patient and his wife have a daughter staying with them for three weeks to assist with the patient's recovery and function as care giver to her mother. Follow-up telephone call three days postdischarge revealed no complications.

An important geriatric case management function is the evaluation of nursing home patients who may need emergency department treatment or rehospitalization; the geriatric case managers actually do on-site evaluations at the nursing home. As a result, unnecessary trips to the emergency department or hospital are avoided, and patient dislocation is kept to a minimum.

Important Points

Case management at Friendly Hills has evolved over time and is currently in a stabilization phase. There are no long-range plans to change or modify the

Figure 6-2. (Continued)

Exercise 2: Did the patient and his wife meet the goals defined in exercise 1? What outcomes were achieved in terms of cost-effectiveness and quality of services? Where do the patient and his wife now access the system on the continuum of care? What are the goals at this point? What tools/resources can be mobilized to assist with the transition to the next access point on the continuum?

A. H. was discovered to have a sternal wound infection on his post-op visit to the LLUMC cardiac surgeon. The patient was afebrile with no obvious wound drainage; however, the sternum was unstable on palpation. The patient was admitted to LLUMC and required intravenous antibiotics, surgical wound debridement with plastic surgery reconstruction of the sternum, and multiple dressing changes with wound care.

Exercise 3: Were the goals defined in exercise 2 realized? At what access point on the continuum is the patient now located? What are the goals at this point? What tools/resources can be mobilized to assist with the transition to another access point?

The patient was sent home with intravenous antibiotics and home health care on hospital day 10 (POD 7). An extensive home teaching plan was developed in conjunction with home health, clinical nurse specialist, LLUMC case manager, physicians at LLUMC and FHHN, and FHHN wound care nurse in order to prepare the patient, wife, and daughter to manage the patient's care. Follow-up visits were coordinated with LLUMC and FHHN physicians, along with managed care department. The patient's daughter extended her visit for two weeks, then arranged for hired assistance after she returned home. With extensive teaching and preparation, the wife and daughter successfully assumed care of the dressings and intravenous antibiotics. Home health visits diminished from three times daily, to once daily for three days, to once weekly. Home health was discontinued altogether after the third week postdischarge when intravenous antibiotics were completed. The patient visited the wound care nurse twice weekly when antibiotics were discontinued for wound evaluation and to reinforce teaching.

Exercise 4: Were the goals defined in exercise 3 realized? What were the outcomes in terms of cost-effectiveness and quality of care? What are the goals in terms of moving the patient along the continuum at this point? What tools/resources could be utilized?

Figure 6-3. Elective Coronary Artery Bypass Surgery Clinical Path

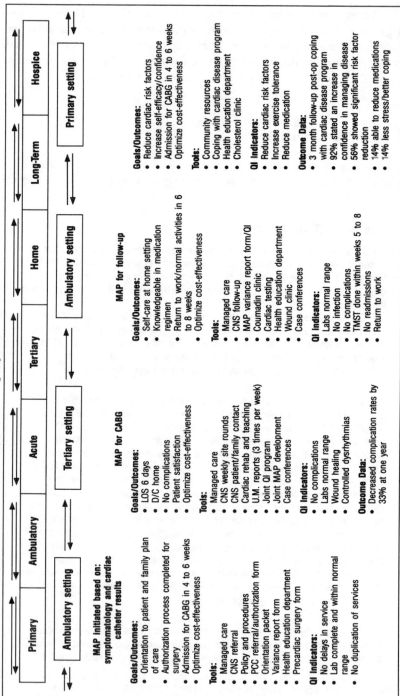

Source: Reprinted, with permission, from Friendly Hills HealthCare Network, La Habra, CA, copyright 1994.

program, but there is a definite willingness to use the program to accommodate unforeseen needs that arise in the system. The following important conclusions have been arrived at from the Friendly Hills case management experience:

- Case management that is ambulatory based is well in tune with the overall shift of care out of the hospital setting.
- Case managers who are responsible for the clinical *and* financial management of enrollees need advanced skills to do their jobs.
- Depending on the organizational setting, change may be most effective when implemented subtly rather than announced publicly.

Chapter Seven

Community-Focused Nurse Case Management at Carondelet St. Mary's Hospital and Health Center

Community-focused nurse case management at Carondelet St. Mary's Hospital and Health Center in Tucson, Arizona, is highly innovative. Nurse case managers provide and coordinate care in an ambulatory setting of 15 community health centers. They use their judgment and experience, not rigid formulas, to determine which patients are most likely to benefit from case management services. Keys to the case manager–client relationships are collaboration and client choice. Well positioned to manage under capitation, the nurse case management network has experience under a Medicare risk contract.

Chapter 7 is divided into the following major sections:

- Background
- Program design, evolution, and goals
- Target population
- Case manager–client relationships (philosophy and practice)
- Activities of case management
- Measurement of success
- Development of capitated nursing HMO reimbursement
- Important points

Background

In response to the shift to prospective payment and resulting decrease in length of stay, Carondelet St. Mary's Hospital and Health Center developed a community-focused nurse case management program. Under the leadership of the vice-president, patient care services, the organization established a unique network structure involving nurses as both coordinators and providers of care.

Information for Chapter 7 was provided by Phyllis Ethridge, M.S.N., R.N., F.A.A.N. (vice-president, patient care services); Cathy Michaels, R.N., Ph.D. (professional nurse case manager and clinical director of research); and Carol D. Falk, M.S., R.N. (professional nurse case manager and president, Carondelet St. Mary's Nursing Enterprise).

Philosophically, the program emphasizes patient/client involvement in care planning and implementation, rather than provider-determined treatment. At its current stage in development, case management addresses the total continuum of care, ranging from health education/prevention to community-based options for care.

Program Design, Evolution, and Goals

When nurse case management began in 1985, nurses on the inpatient units continued to care for patients once they were discharged home. The original design was altered when it became evident that some acute care nurses lacked the knowledge and abilities to project care needs over time and to deal with reimbursement issues. Those nurses with a B.S.N. and community health background were better able to do the job than those with other backgrounds and experience.

The redesigned program features a professional nurse case manager as the hub of a nursing network (see figure 7-1). Nurses in the network function as a group practice, and depending on the particular contract, the nurse case manager may coordinate the services of nursing specialists for acute care, cardiac rehabilitation, hospice, diabetes, private services, ambulatory care, infusion, pulmonary rehabilitation, skilled nursing, community nurse education, and home health. The vice-president of patient care services to whom the network reports is also a member of the group.

The program has three goals: improved quality, improved access, and reduced cost. With respect to *quality*, the process is client-focused, and it strives to enhance the quality of both care and life. Services are matched to individual needs; the program is distinguished by absence of a formula approach for the provision of services. With respect to *access*, the nurse case managers work to maximize access, enhance continuity of care among different providers, and achieve appropriate resource utilization. The *cost reduction* goal encompasses cost-effectiveness, movement from an illness to a health/wellness model, and provision of a continuum of care.

Carondelet has targeted those segments of the client population that can best benefit from nurse case management. This approach differs from that taken by other organizations that use practice guidelines and other tools to determine the appropriateness of case management. The three groups of clients on which Carondelet concentrates are (1) patients with chronic illness, (2) acute care patients whose conditions have been exacerbated by chronic conditions and who will ultimately return to baseline functioning, and (3) patients facing end of life.

Referrals come to the nurse case managers from any part of the Carondelet system, although most come from the acute care staff. The process of deciding who can benefit the most from case management has been a learning experience. Over time, it has become clear that case management services are most effective for patients meeting the following criteria: high recidivism rates;

Figure 7-1. Community-Focused Nurse Case Management Network, Carondelet St. Mary's Hospital and Health Center

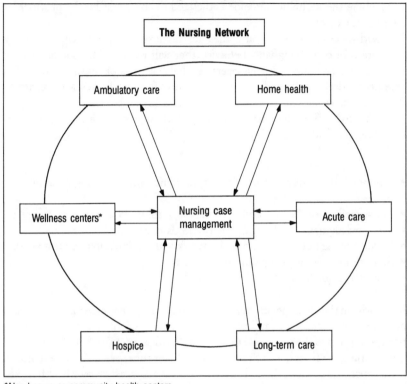

The Nursing Network

Ambulatory care

Home health

Wellness centers*

Nursing case management

Acute care

Hospice

Long-term care

*Also known as community health centers.

Source: Reprinted, with permission, from Carondelet St. Mary's Hospital and Health Center, Tucson, AZ, copyright 1994.

medically complex problems; frailty; chronic illness; terminal illness; cost and/or length-of-stay outliers; cognitive impairment; emotional challenges; inadequate family support; and a high probability of sudden physiologic imbalance requiring frequent emergency department and hospital use.

Application of the criteria is subjective. For example, a client would not have to live alone to qualify on the basis of inadequate family support. If a spouse or child who lived with the client is unable to provide care, the situation would meet the test.

Case Manager–Client Relationships

The nurse case managers work with clients in ways that differ from traditional methods in that they involve collaboration, choice, and patterns. The *collaborative* effort involves the establishment of an initial partnership between client and nurse. Clients are intimately involved in the goal-setting process, unlike systems where the desirable outcome is dictated to the client by the provider or coordinator of care.

With respect to *choice*, outcomes are client-selected, with clients having the option of complying with behavior that will result in the outcomes they have chosen. The nurse case managers also help clients look at *patterns* of health care needs, decisions, choices, utilization, and life-style choices with regard to their health.

Underlying the collaboration-choice-pattern approach is a clear philosophy regarding the following issues:

* Respect for client choices
* Emphasis on client responsibility for outcomes and nurse responsibility for process
* Nurse facilitation (as opposed to doing for or taking over); continuity of care
* Acknowledgment of changing client needs over time
* Linkage of the nurse case manager network with multidisciplinary team efforts
* Shift from hospital to health center focus
* Impact on quality and cost

In a study on the client perspective of working with a nurse case manager, Lamb and Stempel describe the multiple phases that many clients experience, ranging from perception of the nurse case manager as "insider-expert," to bonding, to working, to changing (Lamb and Stempel 1994). Over time, when the case management process takes effect, clients learn new ways to manage their own health needs.

Activities of Case Management

The nurse case managers take six steps to perform their jobs. These are referral; screening to determine client needs; assessment/collaboration; development of a care plan; coordination of services, including working closely with family; and reassessment/evaluation.

Referral, screening, assessment, and plan development are generally done in the hospital, and the coordination of services is done in the community. As a rule of thumb, for new clients or for current clients with new problems, for every hour spent in the home the case manager spends another two to three hours brokering.

Measurement of Success

Carondelet has measured the success of its nurse case management program in several ways. These include client satisfaction, reduction in hospital admission and emergency department visits, decreased costs and acuity of hospital stay, minimization of loss of hospital revenue, increased job satisfaction, and decreased job stress for nurses.

Development of Capitated Nursing HMO Reimbursement

After Carondelet developed its nurse case management program, it successfully developed a method for obtaining reimbursement for services provided to high-risk Medicare recipients enrolled in an HMO. The capitation payment covered not only nurse case management, but also Medicare home health, respite care, and home infusion therapy. The original capitation did not cover community-based care. Patients were referred to the nurse case managers primarily by the hospital but also by staff and contracted physicians in the HMO.

The original capitation arrangement lasted for one and one-half years, and when the contract was renegotiated the capitation arrangement changed in two important ways. First, the community health centers were included under the new capitation arrangement. Also, the capitation payment went directly to the hospital, not to the nursing enterprise—thus involving the entire system in the management of care under capitation. Both of these changes had a positive impact on the nurse case management efforts. The decision of the HMO to establish its own home care agency had a negative impact on nurse case management and at times disrupted the continuum of care that had already been developed. When the capitation contract comes up for renegotiation, Carondelet's nurse case management program hopes to implement new systems for screening risk at the time of enrollment and providing intervention for those most likely to benefit.

Important Points

Over time, Carondelet St. Mary's nurse case management program has evolved and grown. Important points are listed below.

- Develop a method for identifying those clients most likely to benefit from the intervention of case management.
- Focus on interpersonal collaboration between nurse case manager and client.
- Incorporate case management into capitation contracts as a method for co-ordinating care.
- Consider development of case management as a separate business enterprise.

References and Bibliography

Ethridge, P. A nursing HMO: Carondelet St. Mary's experience. *Nursing Management* 22(7):22–27, July 1991.

Ethridge, P. Professional nursing case management improves quality, access and costs. *Nursing Management* 20(3):30–35, Mar. 1989.

Falk, C. Community-based nurse case management. Presentation, New England Health Care Assembly, Boston, Mar. 30, 1994.

Lamb, G. S., and Stempel, J. E. Nurse case management from the client's view: growing as insider-expert. *Nursing Outlook* 42(1):7–13, Jan.–Feb. 1994.

Michaels, C. Carondelet St. Mary's nursing enterprise. *Nursing Clinics of North America* 27(1):77–85, Mar. 1992.

Newman, M., Lamb, G. S., and Michaels, C. Nurse case management, the coming together of theory and practice. *Nursing and Health Care* 12(8):404–8, Oct. 1991.

Chapter Eight

Three Levels of Case Management at Sharp HealthCare

Sharp HealthCare is a sophisticated integrated financing and delivery system including 1,100 physicians, 5 hospitals, 15 clinics, 7 group practices, a home health agency, 3 skilled nursing facilities, related ancillary services, and a wholly owned insurance product (Sharp HealthCare 1993b). System services are accessible to residents of San Diego and Riverside counties in southern California. The Sharp system actively provides care for more than 800,000 patients and over 200,000 HMO covered lives. It is both a Medicare and Medi-Cal provider.

Case management is a key component of integrated care at Sharp, and the system is working with case managers at three different points in the continuum of care. An important feature of case management is its continuing evolution. Case management in 1995 is not the same as case management in 1994, and reshaping of the concept will never be finished.

Chapter 8 is divided into the following main sections:

• System overview
• History and description of case management
• Methods of targeting appropriate enrollees
• The CNS as trauma case manager (an example)
• Future challenges
• Important points

System Overview

Sharp's overall system goal is to manage enrollees' health as well as illness, and to deal with health improvement and access to services *before* illness becomes acute. As a managed care leader, Sharp offers the following (Sharp HealthCare 1993a):

Information for this chapter was provided by Jan Cetti (senior vice-president, quality and mission) and Judy Fix, R.N. (chief operating officer, Sharp Memorial Hospital).

- *Convenience:* The Sharp network is extensive, maximizing patient/member access. Most care is provided by physicians in their offices and in other outpatient locations. A countywide urgent care system ensures immediate access for managed care patients.
- *Continuum of care:* Sharp programs and services include prevention and wellness, acute inpatient care with specialty centers of excellence, rehabilitation, and nursing care. Patients move along the continuum of care, and the system can "bundle" services and offer payers fixed package rates.
- *Continuous quality improvement:* Continuous quality improvement and the development of measurable outcomes is a systemwide priority. Major efforts are in place to define and measure clinical excellence and to use information to educate clinicians. An electronic patient-focused medical record is accessible throughout the system. Clinical leaders are developing quality outcome measures and refining clinical pathways. The system participates in three major national studies to assess its strengths.
- *Contract negotiation:* The Sharp system negotiates on behalf of its multiple providers and entities, and it offers local and national payers competitive arrangements. The Sharp HMO is offered to employers throughout the county.
- *Wellness and prevention:* Sharp emphasizes health and wellness, focusing on health maintenance and prevention.
- *Cost savings:* Both centralized financial planning and purchasing have enabled Sharp to generate significant cost savings.
- *Universal access:* As a supporter of universal access at the most appropriate level of care, Sharp provides a significant amount of charitable care as well as financial support of other institutions that provide care to the indigent. The family practice residency program trains primary care physicians.

History and Description of Case Management Program

At Sharp, case management is the process used to "integrate, coordinate, and advocate for patients requiring extensive services" (Reigel and others 1993). As the system continues to evolve and change, so does case management.

Historically, case management existed at Sharp Memorial Hospital prior to the integration of the system components. The earlier program was the starting point for the development of a more comprehensive model that involves the use of case management at three different points along the continuum of care. At all three points, as described following, nurses perform (or will perform) the role of case manager, with enrollees/patients as the focus.

- *Primary care on an ongoing basis:* Nurses trained in prevention and wellness are responsible for making sure that enrollees have access to health care and periodic health screening. They offer assistance to primary care providers and provide services to enrollees in a variety of settings, including physicians' offices, clinics, businesses, or home settings. The prevention and wellness nurses are responsible for a large enrollee population.

• *Intermediate care*: At the intermediate level of care, nurse practitioners and other staff focus on enrollees with an acute or chronic diagnosis. They may be assigned to ensure that access to care is timely, and that care is delivered according to clinical maps for treatment and resource use. The scope of responsibility includes the acute episode as well as the events prior to and following that event.

The nurse "case managers" at the intermediate level of care combine the roles of utilization review, discharge planning, social service, and quality management. Furthermore, they ensure quality and continuity of care by following patients from the hospital to the home setting. They do not provide direct patient care.

• *Hospital-based specialty case managers*: These case managers focus on the 10 to 15 percent of hospitalized enrollees whose cases cannot be managed by a clinical map. Working closely with physicians and with hospital staff organized along service lines, they report to the service-line administrators and have a dotted-line reporting relationship to the service-line medical directors.

Methods of Targeting Appropriate Enrollees

To determine whether enrollees can benefit from primary care case management, Sharp uses its ongoing health status and risk tracking system, including the following tools: health status questionnaire (formerly SF-36); health risk analysis; risk modification programs; standard preventive guidelines; protocols for managing health; health education; member education; automated data tracking; and standard results reporting.

For enrollees diagnosed with a particular illness, determination of the appropriateness of intermediate level case management is made by using predetermined events or triggers that are built into the managed care IDX information system. If intermediate level case management is needed, the tools used are multidisciplinary clinical maps by diagnostic category; clinical guidelines; automated tracking of actual versus predicted result; monitoring of costs and outcomes; standard results reporting; and reduction in variation/outcomes improvement. Both these tools and those used for primary care case management may be used as appropriate by the hospital-based case managers who handle complicated or compounded clinical conditions.

In some service lines (such as cardiac care), the application of clinical mapping has been so successful that most patients do not need case management. In other service lines (such as oncology), there is a greater need for case management. As care shifts from the inpatient to outpatient setting, the importance of community-based case management has become apparent.

The Clinical Nurse Specialist as Trauma Case Manager

Sharp Memorial, a 415-bed community hospital in the Sharp network, has been a Level II trauma center since 1984. Over 1,100 patients annually are trauma admissions, the result of injury due to falls, motor vehicle accidents, assaults, and violent crimes.

Trauma case management, one of the hospital-based specialty case management roles in the Sharp system, was instituted at the hospital in 1988, when one clinical nurse specialist (CNS) trauma case manager (TCM) provided coverage Monday through Friday. Coverage was increased to seven days per week to accommodate the high volume of trauma patient admissions that occur on weekends. By 1994, the ratio of CNS to case load was on average 1 to 10–15.

The TCM is a key member of the multidisciplinary trauma team. The average case load is 10 to 15 patients, allowing the TCM sufficient time for daily patient assessment, review of clinical status, and family interaction.

Each day, the TCM and medical director of trauma conduct joint rounds on all critically ill trauma patients. Together, they identify high-risk patients by virtue of age, severity of injury, clinical diagnosis, and psychosocial/financial issues. The initial assessment, performed within the first 24 hours of admission, also identifies patients who are potentially high utilizers of resources.

In addition to the joint rounds, the TCM also conducts daily clinical nursing rounds on all trauma patients and participates in weekly multidisciplinary rounds. There is ongoing interaction with the bedside nurse, trauma social worker, family, and medical consultants in order to ensure coordination and continuity of care.

Because trauma is unpredictable, clinical pathways are not used. The TCM's judgment during performance of daily rounds allows for identification of recovery patterns that differ from expectation. The TCM works closely with the care-giving team regarding potential complications.

In carrying out job responsibilities, the TCM serves in a number of roles simultaneously. Among them are educator, consultant, researcher, and manager. These roles are summarized briefly in the following subsections.

Educator Role

The TCM is responsible for teaching the nursing staff who care for trauma patients in the intermediate care and medical/surgical units. Aside from weekly surgical ICU rounds, case studies are often used as teaching devices. On a formal basis, the educational needs of each unit-based CNS are assessed so that training can be provided in a seminar framework.

Consultant Role

The TCM acts as consultant to nursing staff throughout the hospital. As the individual who has worked with the patient and family since admission, the

TCM is able to deal with the stress of reaction to sudden illness and with difficult family dynamics. For example, different ethnic groups may hold particular opinions about the role of heroic efforts. Within a single family, different members may have different views on appropriate treatment. The TCM can work with the family and with clinicians to reach consensus on appropriate care.

Researcher Role

As practitioner and educator, the TCM is in a position to assess trauma patients on a daily basis and to help identify those who deviate from the expected pattern of recovery. On discovery of such deviation from expectation, the TCM can work with the appropriate physician(s) to ensure that the patient's needs are met on a timely basis.

Manager Role

The role of the TCM is not limited to clinical care. Financial resources are a key concern to patient and family, and the TCM becomes involved in this area of care as well. For example, the TCM and discharge planner may work closely together if trauma patients need help with applying for public assistance.

Future Challenges

As Sharp continues to define and operationalize case management as a nursing function, it will address, at a minimum, the following questions:

- How will the role of nurse case managers at various points along the continuum of care affect the existing role of family/primary practice physicians?
- How can the system educate physicians about the importance of advanced practice roles for nurses?
- How can nurses in the system be trained to meet the demands of advanced practice?
- Will state legal and regulatory requirements impede the development of advanced practice roles for nurses?

Important Points

The evolution of case management at Sharp HealthCare suggests that the following points are significant:

- The linkage between hospital-based and community-based case management is important as more and more care is delivered on an outpatient basis.

- Case management depends on clinician support, and the best areas in which to apply the concept are those in which physicians, nurses, and other staff perceive a need and therefore are likely to cooperate.
- Case management is an evolving, not a static, concept.

References and Bibliography

Cerne, F. Engineering a system culture, functioning as a system cultivates integration. *Hospitals and Health Networks* 68(6):36–38, Mar. 20, 1994.

Daleiden, A. L. The CNS as trauma case manager: a new frontier. *Clinical Nurse Specialist* 7(6):295–98, Nov. 6, 1993.

Lumsdon, K. More than revving the engine, systems take tangible steps toward physician and clinical integration. *Hospitals and Health Networks* 68(6):39–43, Mar. 20, 1994.

Riegel, B., Tomlinson, C., Weiss, M., Saks, N., Glancy, M., and Hanley, P. *Sharp Health-Care Manual for Clinical Mapping*, Nov. 1993.

Sharp HealthCare. Press release. Jan. 14, 1993a.

Sharp HealthCare. *Quality Program Blueprint*. Sept. 21, 1993b.

The Transition of Hospital-Based Case Management to System Case Management at Lutheran General

Lutheran General Hospital (LGH) is a teaching, research, and referral hospital located in Park Ridge, Illinois. It is part of Lutheran General Health-System (LGHS), a vertically integrated network of health and human service organizations committed to delivering innovative and comprehensive health care and health-related services to Chicago-area residents.

Case management began at LGH in 1990 under the direction of a case management steering committee. Several years later, the system, LGHS, announced the development of a customer-focused, fully integrated, and seamless continuum of care and designated a Chicagoland Continuum of Care Council to guide the effort. (See figure 9-1.) The goal of the continuum of care effort is to develop a customer-oriented seamless system of services and integrating mechanisms that guides and tracks individuals over time through a comprehensive network of health, medical, and social services, spanning all levels and sites of care and directed toward improving the health status of target populations.

One of the continuum of care implementation teams, the care management continuum team, identified case management as a mechanism to coordinate care and serve as an integrating mechanism. Future case management initiatives at the hospital will become part of the broader scope of care management at the system level.

This chapter is intended to illustrate the way in which system care management can evolve from an initiative that started at one of the system components. In other systems that never developed case management at the component level, the management of care across the continuum may evolve differently and assume more of an ambulatory focus from the outset.

Three people at Lutheran General Hospital/Lutheran General HealthSystem provided information for this chapter: Julie Schaffner, M.S.N., R.N. (vice-president, patient care services); Jeannine Reichert Herbst, B.S.N., R.N. (chairperson, case management operations council); and Wendy Micek, D.N.Sc., R.N. (coordinator of nursing research and special projects). All three have been involved in both hospital case management and in the evolution to system care management.

Figure 9-1. Lutheran General HealthSystem, Chicagoland Continuum of Care Council

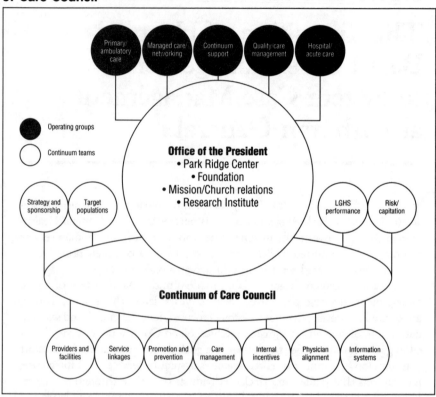

Source: Reprinted, with permission, from Lutheran General HealthSystem, Park Ridge, IL, copyright 1994.

Chapter 9 is divided into the following sections:

- Background
- History and evolution of case management at hospital and system levels
- Program description, organization, and staffing
- Obstacles to developing case management
- Positive factors
- Important points

Background

Lutheran General Hospital (LGH), a 742-bed facility, provides care to 26,000 inpatients and 123,000 outpatients annually. The hospital is a Level I trauma center for children and adults and, as a regional referral center for high-risk pregnancies, it handles approximately 5,000 births annually. Other services offered are comprehensive inpatient and outpatient mental health care, cardiac care, state-of-the-art cancer care, and comprehensive pediatric care provided in a large children's hospital. As the largest independent academic medical center in Illinois, LGH trains 200 residents, 300 medical students, and 170 allied health students annually. Its medical school affiliation is with the University of Chicago Pritzker School of Medicine.

The system of which LGH is a part, Lutheran General HealthSystem (LGHS), was founded in 1897. It is an institution of the Evangelical Lutheran Church in America and is guided by a strong mission, values, and founding philosophy based on human ecology which, as defined in the hospital's "Statement of Philosophy, Values and Mission" is "the understanding and care of human beings as whole persons, in light of their relationships to God, themselves, their families and the society in which they live" (Lutheran General HealthSystem 1993).

The system provides care at more than 74 sites in the Chicago metropolitan area. It has 6,800 associates, more than 800 primary care and subspecialty physicians, and 1,600 volunteers. Lutheran General Medical Group employs 235 physicians, many of whom are primary care physicians. Lutheran General HealthSystem is recognized as an industry leader in the implementation of continuous quality improvement (CQI) initiatives and in the establishment of a comprehensive continuum of care. The system is one of 12 in the country selected by the American Hospital Association as a model system of innovative preparation for health care reform.

The contemporary, interdisciplinary approach to working together is reflected in LGHS's unique organizational design. Specifically, interdependent work groups have been established around major health care trends and system strategic initiatives.

History and Evolution of Case Management at Hospital and System Levels

Case management at LGH began in 1990 with the development of a unit-based program on the geriatric medicine unit. Under the guidance of a case management steering committee, the number of unit-based case management programs grew; some became part of the National Chronic Care Consortium's local geriatric care network program. The hospital moved beyond the unit concept and also established housewide case management initiatives for patients who received care in many different units during their hospital stay.

Unit-based and/or housewide case management was set up in seven clinical areas: orthopedics, psychiatry, cardiovascular surgery, trauma care, medical neurology, neonatology, and respiratory care. Given the differences among the areas, case management varied in structure and focus.

In addition to the unit-based and housewide efforts, LGH has developed case management programs targeted at other specific populations. For example, the hospital provides case management for enrollees of the Lutheran General Health Plan (LGHP), a joint venture of the hospital and the Lutheran General Independent Practice Associates, Inc. The hospital has also begun to extend case management beyond its own boundaries and into the continuum of care.

At the system level, the care management continuum team has begun to look at case management in the broad sense. The group has also begun reviewing methods for identifying high-risk individuals; interdisciplinary assessment teams; applications of clinical management tools (for example, algorithms, protocols, and extended care pathways); and use of a shared information system (for example, clinical data base and patient/client record). A major focus is on patient outcomes.

Although case management activities are performed at both hospital and system levels, the term *case management* is not used with patients and families. Case managers explain their role as coordinators of care, but they deliberately refrain from using a term that is so frequently misunderstood.

Program Description, Organization, and Staffing

Case management at LGH is decentralized and organized around specialty areas. The case managers are coordinators, not direct care givers, who act as client advocates and are responsible for the management of episodes of illness. As care management evolves in a system context, the case managers' role will change, and they will be responsible for improving the health status of a target population. They may become more directly involved in direct patient care as the scope of care expands to include health and wellness activities.

Four years after it had introduced case management, LGH had 10 case managers in place covering the following clinical areas: mental health care, geriatrics, chronic respiratory care, cardiovascular surgery, orthopedics, trauma care, and medical neurology. One case manager was continuum-based and connected with the National Chronic Care Consortium. She was responsible for extended care pathways for older adults and for the linkage of sites of care.

Case managers are a part of the nursing division. Unit-based managers report to a clinical manager (figure 9-2), and those who do housewide case management report directly to a section nursing director (figure 9-3). Given the importance of primary nursing at the hospital, the reporting relationship has facilitated the integration of direct care givers and coordinators. The case managers coordinate the activities of a multidisciplinary team, including not only physicians and primary nurses, but also other professional disciplines.

Initially, the requirements for case managers included a B.S. in nursing and two to three years' experience in a clinical specialty. As the case manager role evolved, so did the requirements for the job. The revised requirements

Figure 9-2.   Lutheran General Hospital's Unit-Based Case Management Model

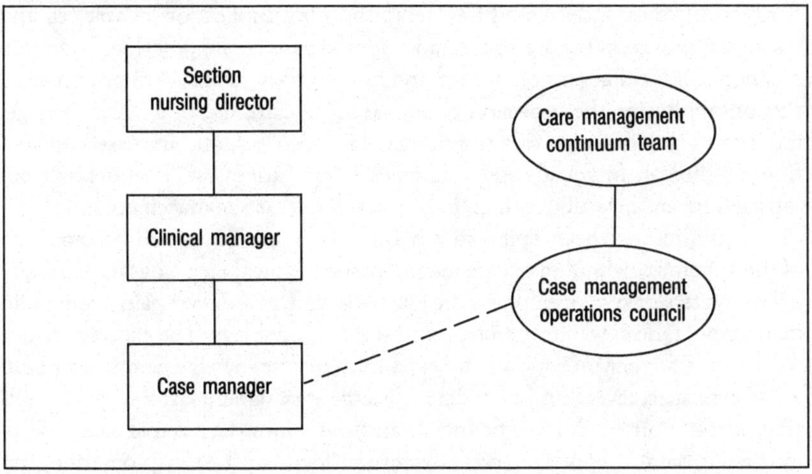

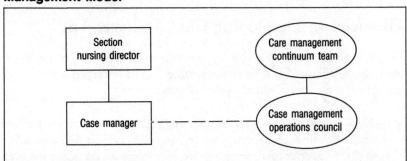

Source: Reprinted, with permission, from Lutheran General HealthSystem, Park Ridge, IL, copyright 1994.

Figure 9-3.   Lutheran General Hospital's Housewide Case Management Model

Source: Reprinted, with permission, from Lutheran General HealthSystem, Park Ridge, IL, copyright 1994.

include an M.S. in nursing, five years of clinical experience in a specialty, and Illinois R.N. licensure. In addition to professional credentialing, case managers need excellent intrapersonal and interpersonal skills, good communication abilities, experience in both individual and group dynamics, and the capability to think proactively. Some of the case managers were recruited from outside the organization, and others came from within the hospital's staff.

The case managers use a number of tools including, but not limited to, clinical protocols and pathways with variance analysis and management, algorithms, and extended care pathways. All case managers have received extensive CQI training.

Although the hospital case management efforts in each clinical specialty vary, in all areas case management has resulted in the following: increased standardization of care; decreased fragmentation and duplication of services and resources; provision of care in the most appropriate setting; increased communication and collaboration in an interdisciplinary team setting; increased accountability for the provision of high-quality care; use of clinical management tools that decrease variation in clinical outcomes; and increased integration of clinical, financial, and outcomes data. Patient, staff, and physician satisfaction are measurably higher as a result of case management.

In the future, the hospital case management initiatives will become part of the system's continuum of care management. Clinical areas that have already been targeted for system emphasis are low back pain, acute chest pain, Coumadin management, deep vein thrombosis, and severe head injury. The expected results will include further integration and expansion of case management to appropriate system sites, levels, and providers; placement of patients in the optimal setting; integration of clinical, financial, and outcomes data across sites; use of integrated data to seek a market advantage; focus on health promotion and illness prevention; increased integration of network services; increased capacity for information systems to support case management; and use of outcomes measures across time and sites of care.

Obstacles to Developing Case Management

During both the initial development and ongoing evolution of case management, both LGH and LGHS have encountered and addressed a number of obstacles. Some are capsulized in the following list.

- *Ambiguity surrounding the need for case management:* The hospital addressed this issue by using comparative data on outcomes and cost to convince the team of the importance of managing care. The information enabled the team to look at LGH's performance from the same perspective that an outside purchaser would have.
- *Ambiguous definition of case management:* Confusion about definition existed at both hospital and system levels. The system has ultimately reached consensus on a definition:

  The service delivered by a provider whose primary responsibility is coordination of care for individuals with complex problems or who are at greater risk. The care is coordinated throughout the episode of illness and across settings. Case management includes assessment, care planning, referral and follow-up that ensures the provision of services according to client need. A case manager acts as a client advocate, monitoring the individual's progress throughout the system (Shaffner 1994).

- *Need for ongoing education:* Both the case managers and everyone with whom they come in contact need ongoing education about their role. For example, new case managers need orientation and training. Existing case managers, who have numerous interactions with clinical and nonclinical people both inside and outside of the organization and whose roles continue to evolve, need ongoing support.
- *Communication:* As case management evolves, so does the need for open and effective communication. The hospital has formed a case management operations council that represents case managers in different specialties and in the continuum of care. The council concentrates on centralizing work efforts as well as on communication across specialty lines.
- *Use of planning and work groups:* In each specialty area, LGH/LGHS uses two groups to plan and implement case management. The design committee is generally the larger group and includes an administrator, a unit medical director, a case manager, and representatives from finance and utilization review. Smaller work teams plan the implementation and include representatives from the design committee, professional staff from the unit, and physicians who admit to the unit.
- *Physician support:* Over time, the importance of support from a unit-based medical director has become clear. This individual helps develop and implement case management and is also key in winning support from other physicians.
- *Inconsistent hospital/physician financial incentives:* Conflicting financial incentives have created problems for case managers who attempt to facilitate the delivery of care. For example, physician reimbursement may encourage increased provision of services while hospital case-based reimbursement may discourage it. At the system level, a physician alignment continuum of care team is addressing some of the issues.
- *Data:* To help case managers function effectively, both within the hospital and across the continuum of care, the hospital/system must provide patient-focused data that are distributed on a regular basis.

Positive Factors

A number of factors have contributed to the initial success and continued growth of case management at both hospital and system levels. They include the following:

- Support from system leadership
- Organizational familiarity and comfort with CQI principles
- Physician interest and support (each clinical area in which case management operates has had a physician "champion")
- Focus on process, not people
- Success of a pilot case management effort before expansion to additional clinical areas

- Existence of coordinated, interdisciplinary treatment teams whose members share common philosophy and vision about patient care
- Collaboration among professional staff and departments
- Ability to interrelate primary nursing with case management
- Dedicated clinical nurse specialists
- Clearly defined and measurable outcomes

Important Points

The LGH/LGHS experience with case/care management at both hospital and system levels offers important suggestions for other providers. These are:

- *Respect the importance of process.* The establishment and evolutionary development of methods for managing care do not happen overnight. Adequate up front time for planning and communication will be well spent.
- *Expect ongoing readjustment of systems and processes implemented.* In line with principles of CQI, case management is evolutionary—it is never "finished."
- *Concentrate on support functions concurrently with the development of case management structure and process.* For example, a computerized patient-focused data base can facilitate access to patient records, help identify a care protocol, and ultimately reduce hospital length of stay.

References and Bibliography

Luthern General HealthSystem. *Statement of Philosophy, Values and Mission.* Park Ridge, IL: LGH, Mar. 1993.

Shaffner, J. Interview with vice president, patient care services, Lutheran General Health-System, Park Ridge, IL, May 12, 1994.

Suggested Curriculum
for Case Managers

Introduction

- Definitions of case management
   Generic, with examples of different models
   System- or organization-specific
- Organizational chart showing how case management relates to system/ organization
- System or organization-specific goals of case management program
- Job description
- Professional issues:
   −Accreditation
   −Compensation
   −Ongoing role assessment, redesign

Background Information

- Environmental factors that require case management approach, such as:
   −National and state health care reform efforts
   −Changing methods of reimbursement
   −Shifting of risk from payers to providers
   −Payer and consumer demands for quality and continuity of care
   −Assumption of responsibility for health and illness of defined population
   −Changing shape of fragmented health care delivery system and potential patient/family confusion
   −Demographic changes (for example, percentage of elderly, uninsured)
- System- or organization-specific justification for case management, such as:
   −Reorganization
   −Reengineering
   −Concern for managed care readiness

Tasks

- Assessment of patient/family: medical, psychosocial, financial needs; support systems

121

- Development of individualized multidisciplinary care plan: goals; plan and contingency plan; consensus/approval; funds/health insurance; legal/ethical issues; allocation of resources; quality issues
- Implementation of plan: coordination; communication
- Monitoring: cost/benefit; satisfaction; adjustment/modification; compliance
- Evaluation of plan

Tools and Techniques (examples)

- Documentation: services; outcomes; time/money/resources/procedures; savings; quality of care
- Clinical paths
- Protocols
- Benchmarking
- Variance analysis

Available Resources

- Computerized patient medical records
- Information systems
- Options for care (for example, nursing homes or home care)

Skill Building

- Role of change agent
- Proactive problem solving
- Performing in an unstructured role
- Telephone techniques
- Courtroom testimony
- Utilization review and documentation
- Discharge planning
- Dealing with health insurance plans: contract compliance; benefits coverage; reporting; coordination with plan staff
- Marketing case management to patients, families, physicians, staff
- Educating patients, families, staff, professional community
- Ensuring senior management support
- Collaboration:
  - Active listening
  - Offering and receiving feedback
  - Dealing with stress, denial, bargaining, anger
  - Handling confrontation
  - Methods for conflict resolution

Appendix B

Researching Various Aspects of Case Management

One way to obtain information on case management programs already in place is to identify concerns specific to your facility and then contact organizations or systems about program features that address those issues.

The examples in this appendix are categorized under 14 broad topics, arranged alphabetically, as follows:

1. Applying case management beyond hospital walls
2. Applying case management in emergency departments
3. Applying case management to Medicare patients
4. Applying case management to outpatient departments
5. Assigning case managers to physicians
6. Beginning case management prior to admission
7. Dealing with advance directives
8. Determining appropriateness of term *case management*
9. Implementing case management at teaching hospitals
10. Involving physicians in case management development
11. Measuring impact of case management
12. Sharing case management with patients and families
13. Shifting from nursing case management to multidisciplinary case management
14. Using management information to measure adherence to clinical paths/ practice guidelines

The information is compiled from the author's direct experience, from personal or telephone interviews, and/or reference in *Hospital Case Management, Including Critical Path Network*, the newsletter published by American Health Consultants, Inc.

For references from the newsletter, the issue date and page numbers are shown in parentheses. Because positions and individuals at the different organizations change frequently, names are not published here. Readers may call the main telephone number listed and ask for the office of the president, chief operating officer, or nursing services to request appropriate direction to case management staff. Appendix D lists the names of individuals and organizations contacted by the author.

Applying Case Management beyond Hospital Walls

Carondelet St. Mary's Hospital and Health Center, Tucson, AZ (602/622-5833) has had a nurse case management network in place since 1985. The target population is elderly and high-risk patients. (Jan. 1993, pp. 14–15, and telephone interview)

Daniel Freeman Memorial Hospital, Inglewood, CA (310/674-7050) goes beyond the hospital walls to deal with outliers and prevent readmissions. (Apr. 1993, pp. 67–68)

The Malden Hospital, Malden, MA (617/322-7560) offers case management consultations both to patients after discharge and also to individuals who have not been hospitalized. The consultation strategy helps the hospital avoid readmissions and other costly procedures. (Author's experience)

At *Vanderbilt University Hospital and Clinic, Nashville, TN (615/322-5000)*, the Center for Patient Care Innovation, funded by a 1990 grant from the Robert Wood Johnson/Pew Charitable Trusts, has developed a patient-focused care model, including case management. For some patients, the case management extends beyond the hospital walls. (Dec. 1993, pp. 209–10, 215)

Applying Case Management in Emergency Departments

DeKalb Medical Center, Decatur, GA (404/501-1000) uses clinical pathways and case management in the emergency department. Examples of successful application are in the treatment of chest pain and rape victims. (Nov. 1993, pp. 200–204)

As a consequence of inpatient case management growth at *The Malden Hospital, Malden, MA (617/322-7560)*, other hospital departments, including the emergency department, requested case management assistance. Case managers assist emergency department staff in linking patients and families to appropriate services and agencies. (Feb. 1994, pp. 31–33)

Applying Case Management to Medicare Patients

Carondelet St. Mary's Hospital and Health Center, Tucson, AZ (602/622-5833) has a unique case manager network and experience with a capitated program for Medicare recipients. (Telephone interview)

St. Peter's Medical Center, New Brunswick, NJ (908/745-8600) provides case management to elderly patients as a group, rather than to patients within particular DRG categories. The case managers are "patient advocates" who deal with both clinical and nonclinical issues. (Jan. 1993, p. 15)

Stanford University Hospital, Stanford, CA (415/723-4000) has a community case manager who coordinates care for enrollees in a capitated Medicare risk HMO. (Telephone interview)

Applying Case Management to Outpatient Departments

Stanford University Hospital, Stanford, CA (415/723-4000) has extended case management into four faculty practice clinics: obstetrics/gynecology, hematology/oncology, pain, and bone marrow transplants. In three of the four clinics, the case managers coordinate outpatient and inpatient care. (Telephone interview)

Assigning Case Managers to Physicians

St. Joseph's Medical Center, Burbank, CA (818/843-5111) assigns its case managers to physician groups (all pulmonologists and all nephrologists, for example). The hospital and physicians prefer this approach to the previous unit-based assignments. (Dec. 1993, pp. 207–8)

With 160 active physicians, *The Malden Hospital* in *Malden, MA (617/322-7560)*, a 200-bed community hospital, has assigned one case manager to each physician or physician group. The system provides a simple contact point for all patient information. (Feb. 1994, pp. 26, 31–33, and author's experience)

HCA Tallahassee Community Hospital, Tallahassee, FL (904/656-5000) has assigned 170 staff physicians to six case managers. The case managers run interference, do discharge planning, and assist physicians in keeping their practices organized. (Feb. 1993, p. 23)

Beginning Case Management Prior to Admission

For elective surgery cases, *Baptist Memorial Hospital, Memphis, TN (901/226-5000)* includes in its case management function patient education in the physician's office. The early patient education is preferable to the previous system, under which education was provided postanesthesia and patients were too drowsy to comprehend the information. (Jan. 1993, p. 3)

Southwest Community Health System and Hospital, Middleburg Heights, OH (216/826-8000) combines three components in its case management program: inpatient, outpatient, and preadmission. For the preadmission part, a registered nurse who works in patient registration deals with patient compliance with acute care criteria, working with physicians on observation bed status where necessary, and facilitating admission to the most appropriate unit. (June, 1993, pp. 114–16)

Dealing with Advance Directives (Often a Stumbling Block to Efficient Delivery of Care)

Baptist Memorial Hospital, Memphis, TN (901/226-5000) puts advance directives directly on what it calls *CARE paths.* (Jan. 1993, p. 3)

The case managers for geriatric patients at *Friendly Hills HealthCare Network, La Habra, CA (310/905-3009)* actively address advance directives issues with patients. (Telephone interview)

Determining Appropriateness of Term *Case Management*

Many organizations find the term *case management* to be misleading and confusing and therefore have come up with other alternatives. *Robert F. Kennedy Medical Center, Hawthorne, CA (310/973-1711)* uses the term *care management.* *Strong Memorial Hospital of the University of Rochester, Rochester, NY (716/275-2644)* uses the term *collaborative care* to describe its multidisciplinary program. (Sept. 1993, pp. 166–68)

Implementing Case Management at Teaching Hospitals

Stanford University Hospital, Stanford, CA (415/723-4000) uses case management in inpatient service lines, in faculty clinics, in the community, and in resident teaching. (Telephone interview)

New England Medical Center, Boston, MA (617/956-5000) was a pioneer with its introduction of nursing case management in the 1980s. In the 1990s, the hospital's efforts have shifted to patient-focused collaborative practice initiatives. (Personal and telephone interviews)

Involving Physicians in Case Management Development

Brighton Medical Center, Portland, ME (207/879-8044) believes that physician involvement in case management is a "sell job," not a "tell job." After a successful 18-month pilot program, the physicians have been very involved in planning for the next phase. (Feb. 1993, pp. 21–22)

The Malden Hospital, Malden, MA (617/322-7560) involved physicians in the case management task force that planned the program and later commissioned IPA physicians to perform hospitalwide utilization management and quality assurance activities for all patients. (Author's experience)

Measuring Impact of Case Management

Beth Israel Medical Center, New York, NY (212/420-2000) received a $150,000 grant from the United Hospital Fund in New York to study the impact of case management on congestive heart failure. The two-year study began in spring 1993. (May 1993, pp. 81–83)

Baptist Memorial Hospital, Memphis, TN (901/226-5000) looks beyond cost as a measure of the impact of case management. The hospital conducts pre-case and post-case management satisfaction surveys for staff, patients, and families. (Nov. 1993, p. 192)

St. Vincent Medical Center, Toledo, OH (419/321-3232) generates quarterly reports on the impact of case management, emphasizing financial reports on cost, not charges. (Nov. 1993, pp. 192–93)

Sharing Case Management with Patients and Their Families

Kennestone Hospital, Marietta, GA (404/793-5000) and Anne Arundel Medical Center, Annapolis, MD (410/267-1000) both display easy-to-understand clinical paths in the patient's room in order to share expectations with patients and their families. (Jan. 1993, pp. 1–2)

Baptist Memorial Hospital, Memphis, TN (901/226-5000) shares information on the expected patient course of action but does not display the actual clinical path because so many patients are exceptions to the rule. (Jan. 1993, pp. 2–3 and telephone interview)

Providence Hospital, Everett, WA (206/258-7123) uses computer graphics to create patient-friendly information on what to expect. The pictures are especially helpful when patients are multilingual. (Aug. 1993, pp. 137–40)

St. Vincent Hospital and Medical Center, Portland, OR (503/297-4411) uses "patient-oriented itineraries" that are written in large print in multiple languages. The itineraries contain medical information on pain and medication, among other topics, and also suggestions for personal care. (Aug. 1993, pp. 141–42)

Shifting from Nursing Case Management to Multidisciplinary Case Management

Alliant Health System, Louisville, KY (502/629-8025) has three hospitals with a total of 1,000 beds. It had modeled its original clinical pathways on New

England Medical Center's nursing case management. Like NEMC, the hospital took a second look at their tools and the lack of physician buy-in. (Mar. 1993, pp. 41–45)

Using Management Information System to Measure Adherence to Clinical Paths/Practical Guidelines

Medicus Systems, Evanston, IL (708/570-7500) developed software that can provide a quick picture of a patient's condition, including input from multiple disciplines. *Lakeland Regional Medical Center in Lakeland, FL (813/687-1100)* was a test site for the software. (Jan. 1993, pp. 6–8)

Carondelet St. Mary's Hospital and Health Center, Tucson, AZ (602/622-5833) computerized data collection and utilization for its Medicare risk project in 1990. (Jan. 1993, p. 6, and telephone interview)

Appendix C

Selecting a Consultant

If your organization decides to use outside consultation to learn more about case management and facilitate program development and implementation, be sure to ask the following questions.

- Does your organization need assistance in developing case management, or does it need operational tuning for a program that is already in place?
- Do you want a conceptual consultant or a user/consultant who has been on both sides of the fence and can offer helpful suggestions from personal experience?
- Is the consultant's approach to case management a standard one (for example, nursing case management), or does it vary according to the politics, resources, and preferences of the client?
- What is the consultant's approach to involvement of physicians and other clinicians and administrative staff in the design and implementation phases?
- Does the consultant have experience in organizations similar to yours (for example, community or teaching hospital, or network)?
- Do you need/want ongoing technical assistance, or do you want help only during start-up?

Appendix D

Resource Guide

Organization	Contacts
Baptist Hospital Memphis, TN	Jamie Patterson, R.N., M.S.N., M.B.A.
Beverly Hospital Beverly, MA	Robert Fanning Jeanne M. Holland
Carondelet St. Mary's Hospital and Health Center Tucson, AZ	Carol D. Falk, M.S., R.N. Cathy Michaels, R.N., Ph.D.
The Center for Case Management Natick, MA	Karen Zander, R.N., M.S., C.S.
Community Medical Alliance Boston, MA	David L. Rosenbloom
Franklin Health Group Ramsey, NJ	David Levy, M.D. David J. Hines
Friendly Hills HealthCare Network La Habra, CA	Nancy Brown, R.N. Alison Jacoby, R.N., M.S.N. Lynn Mumaw, Geriatric Nurse Practitioner
General Electric Aircraft Engines Lynn, MA	Robert S. Galvin, M.D.
Health Care Spectrum Inc. Marblehead, MA	Andrew H. Nighswander
Healthfront VHA Woburn, MA	Kelly Breazeale
Sue Keener Associates Arlington Heights, IL	Susan B. Keener

Organization	*Contacts*
The Malden Hospital Malden, MA	Lyle G. Bohlman, M.D. Stanley J. Krygowski Richard A. Hochman, M.D. Evelyn M. Soldano, R.N., M.A., C.C.M.
McDermott, Will and Emery Boston, MA	Harvey W. Freishtat, Esq.
New England Medical Center Boston, MA	Mary Lou Salome Etheredge, R.N., M.S. Jerome H. Grossman, M.D.
Phoenix Health Plan Phoenix, AZ	Naim Munir, M.D.
Ropes and Gray Boston, MA	Michael Christensen
Salem Hospital Salem, MA	Frank P. Morse, M.D. Neil S. Shore, M.D. David Wright, Esq.
Sharp HealthCare San Diego, CA	Jan Cetti Judy Fix, R.N.
Stanford University Hospital Stanford, CA	Cindy Day, R.N., M.S.
Winchester Medical Center Winchester, VA	Lisa Zerull, R.N., B.S.N.

Index

(continued)

Additional Books of Interest

Outpatient Case Management: Strategies for a New Reality
edited by Michelle Regan Donovan and Theodore A. Matson

Outpatient Case Management presents a framework for implementing case management strategies in the outpatient arena. This book provides general guidelines on case management and underscores the importance of this tool in a changing health care delivery system. In-depth discussions cover: the planning agenda, needs assessment, and other special considerations for developing case management programs; building strong working relationships with private payers; creating a seamless continuum of care, comprehensive care planning, and communications between inpatient and outpatient service providers; and the role and function of the case manager, including cost control responsibilities. Sixteen specific examples of different successful programs of all types across the country are presented.

Catalog No. E99-027100 (must be included when ordering)
1994. 298 pages, 20 figures, 8 tables.
$58.95 (AHA members, $48.95)

Clinical Paths: Tools for Outcomes Management
edited by Patrice L. Spath

This groundbreaking book explores the major strategy issues related to the development and implementation of clinical paths. These issues include the relationship between clinical paths and case management, the use of clinical paths to document patient care (and the legal ramifications of such a decision), and how path-based care can promote improvements in patient treatment. Ways clinicians use these paths to decrease variation in patient care, reduce system confusion, and improve communication and collaboration among caregivers are also discussed. This book presents case studies of ten organizations and their experiences with developing and implementing clinical paths.

Catalog No. E99-027101 (must be included when ordering)
1994. 288 pages, 101 figures, 3 tables.
$59.95 (AHA members, $49.95)

To order, call TOLL FREE
1-800-AHA-2626